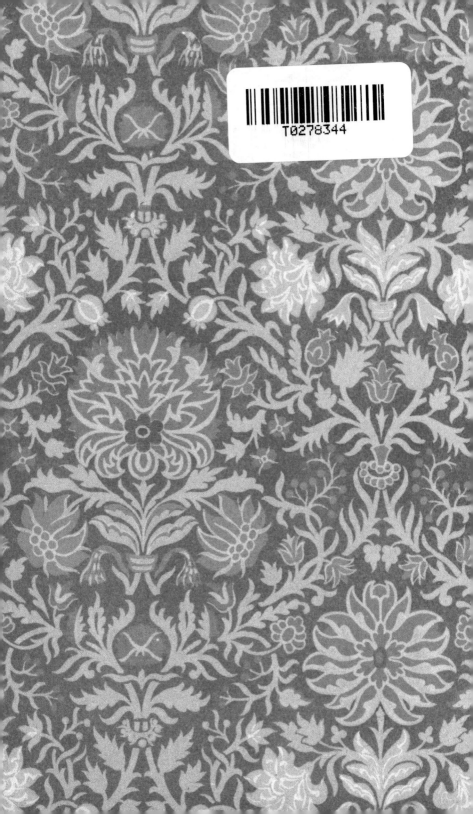

ANDREAS VESALIUS

☙ Books in the RENAISSANCE LIVES series explore and illustrate the life histories and achievements of significant artists, rulers, intellectuals and scientists in the early modern world. They delve into literature, philosophy, the history of art, science and natural history and cover narratives of exploration, statecraft and technology.

Series Editor: François Quiviger

ANDREAS VESALIUS

Anatomy and the World of Books

SACHIKO KUSUKAWA

REAKTION BOOKS

In memory of Toru Kusukawa

Published by Reaktion Books Ltd
Unit 32, Waterside
44–48 Wharf Road
London N1 7UX, UK
www.reaktionbooks.co.uk

First published 2024

Printed and bound in India by Replika Press Pvt. Ltd

A catalogue record for this book is available from the British Library

ISBN 978 1 78914 852 7

COVER: Hand-coloured portrait of Andreas Vesalius, from *De humani corporis fabrica* (Basel, 1543). Photo Universitätsbibliothek Basel (UBH AN I 15).

CONTENTS

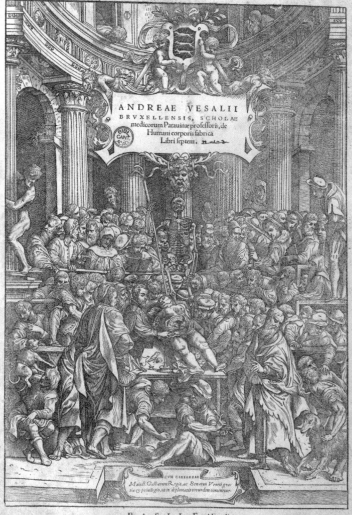

ANDREAE VESALII
BRVXELLENSIS, SCHOLAE
medicorum Patauinæ professoris, de
Humani corporis fabrica
Libri septem.

CVM CAESAREAE
Maiest. Galliarum Regis, ac Senatus Veneti gratia & priuilegio, ut in diplomatis eorundem continetur.

BASILEAE.

Introduction

his frontispiece is the most iconic in the history of medicine (illus. 1). In the plaque at the top, the title of the book and its author are announced in Latin, the academic language of the time. Translated, it reads: 'By Andreas Vesalius of Brussels, Professor of the Paduan School of Physicians, Seven Books about the Fabric of the Human Body.' Andreas Vesalius was the Latinized name of Andries van Wesel (1514–1564), a young man in a hurry. It is no accident that his name is the most visible, in the largest capital letters on the first line. His family, the Wijtincks, originated in Wesel, 50 kilometres (31 mi.) north of Düsseldorf.[1] Wesel in Low German means weasel, and the shield held by two naked boys (or putti) above the plaque shows three of them in the coat of arms of Vesalius's family. The phrase 'fabric of the human body' – meaning the anatomical structure of the human body – was not new. There was an earlier publication with the same title summarizing the views of Galen of Pergamum, a Greek physician who worked in second-century Rome and a major authority in European academic medicine since the Middle Ages. But it is Vesalius's book that is now known by the Latin name *Fabrica*.

The book was an elaborate job application. It opened with a letter addressed to the 'divine, the mightiest and the most un-vanquished' Holy Roman Emperor, Charles V (1500–1558).[2] Soon after presenting a copy of *Fabrica* to Charles, Vesalius was

1 Frontispiece of Vesalius, *De humani corporis fabrica* (1543). Its page height is 43 centimetres/17 in., namely double the height of this page.

appointed one of his physicians. The book made Vesalius's career and defined his reputation. The following pages are about this large and beautiful book that was carefully designed to present anatomical knowledge based on first-hand dissection.

A professor of medicine who urged his peers and students to dissect the human body with their own hands might well deserve praise for heroism if human dissection had been banned at the time. But, as the historian Katharine Park and others have repeatedly pointed out, human dissection was not prohibited by the Catholic Church.[3] Along with the myth that people believed the world was flat until Columbus's voyage, this is one of the common and enduring misconceptions in history of science. From the late thirteenth century, autopsies had been carried out when foul play was suspected. By 1316, the University of Bologna instituted a 'public anatomy', an annual dissection of a human cadaver for medical students. The University of Montpellier followed suit by 1340, as did the Universities of Padua and Paris soon afterwards. By the beginning of the sixteenth century, statutory provision of an annual anatomy had become standard for medical faculties, at least on paper.[4]

However, as Vesalius lamented in his address to the emperor, the medical schools were doing it all wrong: those expounding the body from written descriptions no longer dissected the body as the ancient Greeks had done, and those tasked with the dissection were too unlettered to explain what they were dissecting.[5] In ancient Greece, there had been a unity to the art of healing based on regimen (regulating daily routines such as diet and exercise), medication and surgery, all of which required a hands-on approach. After the Roman Empire fell to the Goths, this unity fell apart. European physicians came to see these fields as beneath their dignity because they involved the use of their hands, and relegated them to apothecaries, barbers or servants, who in turn had no idea or appreciation of the work of the ancients. The loss of surgical competence further led to a 'disastrous shipwreck' for the study of anatomy when – because it was a significant part of natural philosophy – anatomy should have been studied avidly as the bedrock of medicine.

Vesalius was writing these words soon after the rediscovery of important anatomical works by Galen, especially *On Anatomical Procedures*, which revealed Galen's own commitment to first-hand dissection. Rather than something brand new that he was the first to advocate, first-hand dissection was a classical approach that Vesalius was eager to revive and emulate. Thanks to the emperor's support, Vesalius acknowledged, all studies, including medicine, were now coming back to life again. In turn, Vesalius pledged to play his part by bringing the knowledge of human anatomy back from the dead.

Vesalius wrote in the language and style typical of the Renaissance – a time when reviving past achievements of ancient Greece or Rome was a way to contribute to knowledge and scholarship of the present. Historians call this preoccupation with classical culture 'humanism' (not to be confused with its modern sense of non-religious, secular human values) after the scholars and teachers in Italy who promoted the study of humanities as advocated by classical authors such as the Roman orator Cicero (106–43 BCE). Since the fifteenth century, these humanists had been interested in the recovery, restoration and emulation of classical culture, which in turn lent authority and credibility to their views. Armed with proficiency in Latin and some Greek, they hunted for manuscripts in libraries across Europe and pored over inscriptions on ancient coins and ruins. Their newly edited Greek texts and Latin translations made afresh from such Greek editions were better, they claimed, than the earlier Arabic versions on which much of European academic knowledge had been founded. Humanists made a deliberate effort to break away from their immediate past by harking back to a more distant and glorious period. They visibly marked their difference by adopting the lettering style of older manuscripts and ancient monuments.[6] In the dedications of their works to the elite from whom they hoped to obtain gainful employment, it became a trope for humanists to credit their patrons with halting the decline of civilization by supporting the recovery of classical culture and learning.

By the time Vesalius was penning his letter to the emperor, many such dedications had been written to flatter an actual or hoped-for patron. With a remarkable sense of self-awareness, Vesalius condemned this 'hackneyed ritual' that showered on anybody indiscriminate praise such as 'admirable learning, singular prudence, remarkable clemency, keen judgement, untiring generosity'.[7] And yet it was obvious, Vesalius declared, that the emperor exceeded any mortal in all of these virtues. Condemning others as flatterers in order to present oneself as telling the truth was in itself a rhetorical move. Throughout his book, Vesalius made effective use of classical rhetoric and tropes to make his points.

Humanist culture is thus associated with texts, books and libraries, but it also had material and aesthetic dimensions. Princely and noble collectors, especially in Rome, began acquiring sculptures unearthed from ancient sites and from the fifteenth century displayed them in their homes, gardens and museums.[8] It became a rite of passage for artists to visit Rome and capture what was left of the glorious classical past amid ruins and vegetation. An early such visitor from the Netherlands was the painter Maarten van Heemskerck, who made several drawings of ruins and sculptures, one of which was of a seated classical figure missing its arms and legs displayed in the Belvedere Courtyard at the Vatican (illus. 2).[9] Such drawings became the basis of artistic creations or of studying styles of classical architecture.[10]

Vesalius benefited from the work of artists who were fluent in the classicizing trends of the period. For instance, the fluted columns with acanthus leaf capitals in the frontispiece (illus. 1)

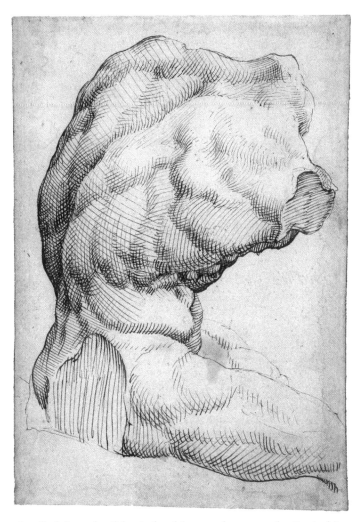

signalled the style of classical architecture known as the Corinthian order. The curvature of the structure above the columns hinted at a circular space reminiscent of a pantheon-like edifice. This composition was not just for displaying the classicizing taste of the period, however. According to Vesalius, the frontispiece

2 Study of the Belvedere Torso by Maarten van Heemskerck, *c.* 1532–6, ink on paper, 18.7 × 13.4 centimetres/7⅓ × 5¼ in.

showed half of the circular type of setting used in his public anatomies in Bologna and Padua.[11] He was referring to the wooden scaffold rather than the architectural setting itself, since there was no corresponding classical building in Bologna or Padua like the one depicted in the frontispiece. This was a scene of a fictional, idealized theatre, not a record of what Vesalius's dissection actually looked like.

A theatre, as Vesalius noted, was a space large enough to accommodate spectators, and the frontispiece shows them crammed, several rows deep, along a stepped wooden structure with some seating.[12] Among a motley gathering of onlookers is a man standing on a ledge at the right-hand edge as if to get a better view of the dissection. He is wearing a beret, fur-trimmed coat and slashed hose, the height of fashionability.[13] He is counterbalanced by a naked male figure to the far left, clinging on to a column, similarly looking down on the dissection. Such a contrast of clothed and unclothed figures was a well-known form of artistic counterpoise.[14] It also draws attention to the stark contrast between life and death in the anatomy theatre.

In the uppermost tier of spectators, figures at the far left and the far right point to the centre of the scene where there is a skeleton holding a stand. The stand was probably the kind of support on which Vesalius placed an articulated skeleton – he brought one to his public anatomy so that he could begin by describing the bones before dissecting the body. Some of the spectators look young as they don't have beards (considered a mark of maturity at the time); others are bearded and/or bald, or show lines on their faces, and appear older. Several are watching intently, leaning forward; some are conversing with each other, and a few appear to have brought books with them. Vesalius had an ambivalent relationship with his spectators – they could be frustratingly unresponsive to his ideas, but he also hoped to co-opt them as witnesses to his work.

Also present in the theatre are figures in cowls, indicating members of a mendicant order. One of them is shown in profile seated at the feet of the fashionable young man at the edge of the scene. At Padua, the mendicants dominated the teaching of theology, and Vesalius wryly remarked that theologians were 'present in great numbers as spectators when we dissect the organs of generation in the schools'.[15] In front of the hooded figure is another bearded figure holding a magnifying glass to his left eye (illus. 5). And in the row in front of him, diagonally below, we can spot the head of a man with spectacles. A magnifying glass could be used as a reading glass in the period, and spectacles were in circulation in Europe by the late thirteenth century.[16] It is unlikely that such optical instruments would have helped spectators from the distance represented in the frontispiece to see any better the dissected body in the centre of the theatre. Nor does Vesalius state that he used magnifying glasses for his observation, though he did note that the crystalline humour (lens) in the eye, when held on the tip of a knife over a piece of paper with writing, made the letters appear larger 'like a magnifying glass'.[17] The figures with sight-enhancing instruments help express a more general point about paying attention to details, which is what Vesalius expected of the readers of his book.

In the centre of the theatre, underneath the skeleton, a male figure stands at the dissection table with one hand pointing upwards, and the other hand with a knife resting on the dissected body. This is Vesalius. On the table are some surgical instruments as well as writing implements, tools that defined Vesalius's identity. The body is that of a woman, a less commonly available subject of public anatomy at the time. The cadaver of the woman may well have evoked an imperial association with the birth of Julius Caesar, believed to have been delivered surgically from his dead mother.[18] In front of the dissection table on the floor is a man with a cap in a somewhat contorted pose who appears to be refusing to hand over a razor to another man. Perhaps he represents the cutters Vesalius had criticized as unlettered. There are three largish figures in the foreground in classical robes and sandals – two to the left of Vesalius, and one across from them who appears to be distracted by a dog held by another person. Counterbalancing the dog, at the opposite side to the far left, a monkey with chains is shown with its keeper.

The classical figures and animals hint at the main features of Vesalius's argument. As a humanist physician, he set out to try and restore comprehensively Galen's project of describing human anatomy based on first-hand dissection. In the process, he discovered that Galen had not always dissected human bodies. This created a challenge for Vesalius in justifying his view of the human body against what Galen and his followers had erroneously described. Vesalius deployed his humanist training to explain some of the errors as resulting from confused terminology and vagaries of manuscript transmission, but the point he made most frequently was that Galen had not dissected a human body. Galen's descriptions better fitted the anatomy of dogs and monkeys.

At the time of publication, a full-page pictorial frontispiece such as *Fabrica*'s was rare, not just for scientific books, but for any printed book. Time-consuming and expensive, it made an important statement about the author and his work. It was also used in the companion piece to *Fabrica* called *Epitome of the Seven Books about the Fabric of the Human Body* (illus. 3), dedicated to the son of Charles V, the future Philip II (1527–1598). It was a brief summary of *Fabrica*, with just eleven pages of text and eleven full-page figures, though printed on larger paper. In the letter to Philip, Vesalius repeated the point that anatomy was an important part of natural philosophy that tackled the fabric of 'the most perfect and most worthy creature of all'.[19] Every part of the body was presented succinctly in the book 'like an image' to those

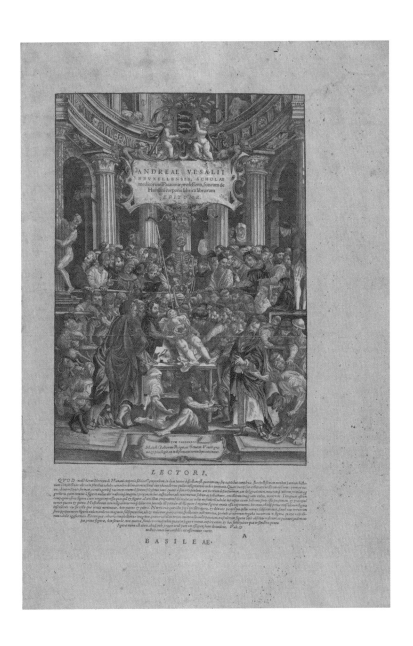

3 Hand-coloured frontispiece of *Epitome* (1543). This copy was once owned by Alexander Macalister (1844–1919), second professor of anatomy at Cambridge. Page height 57 centimetres/22²⁄₅ in.

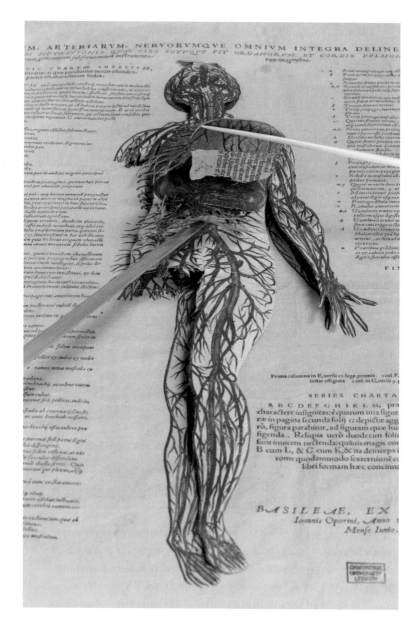

4 Paper manikin, *Epitome* (1543).

studying the work of nature. A striking feature of *Epitome* was its layered manikin composed of paper parts (illus. 4) that readers were expected to construct.

When compared to other recent books on anatomy, *Fabrica* was a large book, and *Epitome* a *very* large one. A page of *Fabrica* is twice the height of this page, and that of *Epitome* just shy of three times this page. In the year of their publication, *Fabrica* (4 florins and 10 batzen) and *Epitome* (4½ batzen) were sold together for just under 5 florins, equivalent to 34 meals in a public house in Basle.[20] *Fabrica* was more expensive than another book published in the same year, Nicolaus Copernicus's *On the Revolutions of the Heavenly Spheres*, priced at 1 florin in 1547. Copernicus's book contained about four hundred smaller pages (page height *c.* 30 centimetres/11⅘ in.) and many fewer illustrations than *Fabrica*, which was almost seven hundred pages long. Given its size and price, *Fabrica* was not a regular textbook that students would have purchased, though *Epitome* would certainly have been more affordable.

Coloured copies would have cost more, but apart from the dedication copy to the emperor, few surviving copies are coloured throughout.[21] One advantage of a coloured copy is that it shows up more vividly the intricate composition of the frontispiece. For example, we can better make out the figure in a white robe (illus. 5) holding a magnifying glass in front of the man in a black cowl, and it also appears as if there are two women at the back between the two columns – one in a white headdress and blue garment and another standing next to her. Vesalius did not mention that any women were present at his dissections, though we know from later accounts that girls attended some of the anatomies at Montpellier.[22]

There is some danger of overreading the frontispiece by trying to identify the actual building or people (apart from Vesalius) depicted in it. While we must accept that it is a fictional scene

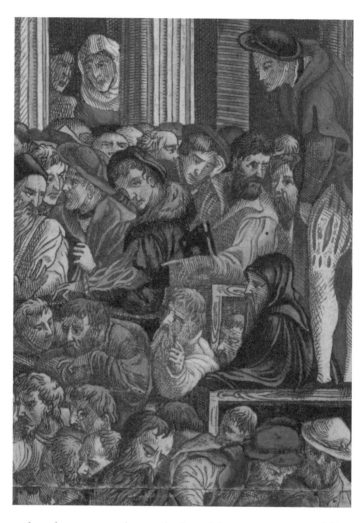

rather than an actual record of a public anatomy, it would be equally wrong to presume that it is a purely decorative piece where the artist had free rein in filling out the page with fashionable classicizing themes. Vesalius pointed his readers to the arches in 'the figure placed at the front of the volume' when

5 Bearded man in a white robe with a magnifying glass and women between the columns, detail of illus. 3.

describing the vertebrae. The twelfth thoracic vertebra did not have parts inserting into either the vertebra above or below it and was simply supported on both ends by other vertebrae, akin to the stone 'between others in vaulted and arched buildings which is supported on each side though it supports no stone itself'.[23] Vesalius thus surmised that it was placed in the middle of the back for stability just like the keystone at the apex of an arch. This is one of the many instances where Vesalius used an analogy with human-made structures to explain the function of a part of the human body. It also highlights an important point, confirmed throughout the book, that Vesalius was closely involved in the design of its illustrations. Images of *Fabrica* were an important part of the book's identity, and I therefore draw extensively on them in the following pages (unless otherwise stated in the captions, illustrations in this book are from *Fabrica* (1543)).

Learned physicians and university professors had worked closely with printers before, but Vesalius exercised unusually close control over the production of the entire book, from the frontispiece, the illustrations, the decorative initials, the type fonts and the use of margins to the paper manikin and the index at the end. Though *Fabrica* is best known for its impressive images, we should not forget that they worked alongside almost 650 pages of text describing the form and function of the parts of the body. The whole book embodied his vision of anatomical knowledge.

Vesalius was not the first to advocate first-hand dissection, teach dissection at university, include illustrations in a book on anatomy, find fault with Galen or dedicate an anatomical book to an emperor. Yet there were some remarkable things about his book. In many ways, a book might seem like a poor medium for promoting first-hand dissection and describing a three-dimensional body. But a book was a symbol of learned medicine, and Vesalius found some ingenious ways to exploit its visual and material dimensions in order to present knowledge about the 'fabric of the human body'.

Fabrica was a Latin word that carried the connotation of something that had been made. Vesalius's book was first and foremost about the structure of the human body – *how it was made*. And in order to find out how the body was made, it was necessary to dissect it. As Vesalius repeated time and again in *Fabrica*, a successful dissection presupposed some knowledge of how that part of the body was made. Dissection was thus a form of *unmaking*. Vesalius wove an intricate connection between the making and unmaking of the human body throughout his book by alternating his descriptions of parts of the body with instructions on how to dissect them.

The word *fabrica* also presupposed a maker, and Vesalius often invoked God as the maker of the human body, especially when defending his disagreements with Galen and others. His gesture in the frontispiece of pointing upwards may well be a reference to this ultimate authority. Between God and the human body, Vesalius is shown as the central figure presenting true knowledge about the human body. He believed that such a knowledge could be conveyed in a printed book.

In order to appreciate why books were central to Vesalius's life, I begin with the world of books that shaped the culture of learned medicine well before his time, and the role of printed books in the careers of authors of anatomical books, several of which were known to Vesalius. In Paris, Vesalius learned that he had a knack for dissection, and watched his teachers publish humanist medical books in handsome fonts. He cut his teeth on the minutiae of book production with his early publications. This experience helped Vesalius design many aspects of his *Fabrica*. Though we do not know for certain the names of the artists for his book, their techniques were harnessed by Vesalius to create images that helped make his points about the human body. I then discuss three major aspects of the book: its relation to the anatomical theatre, the kinds of body presented in it, and Vesalius's own view of himself. The intertwined theme of making and unmaking the body explains how the design and the content of the book formed a unity in expressing 'the fabric of the human body'. Though not all the points Vesalius made were accepted or even noticed by his contemporary readers, his reputation was shaped by his book.

ONE

Learned Medicine and Its Books

niversities – initially meaning a guild of students or teaching masters – had been established since the late twelfth century in Europe. They were institutions through which specialist training was offered to those intending to pursue a career in theology, law or medicine. Based on broadly similar curricula and requirements, university degrees became qualifications recognized across Europe. Central to such a university education were books. The experience of Hartmann Schedel (1440–1514), who went to Padua in the 1460s (more than seventy years before Vesalius arrived there) helpfully illustrates the place of books in academic medicine.[1]

HARTMANN SCHEDEL GOES TO PADUA

When Hartmann Schedel, a merchant's son from Nuremberg, enrolled in the medical faculty of the University of Padua in 1463, he was following in the footsteps of many a student before him who believed that a degree from a renowned university would improve his prospects as a physician. This was also the hope of countless others who came after him, including Vesalius. A degree from the arts faculty was required before studying medicine and many foreign students, including Schedel, obtained their arts degree closer to home before travelling to Italy.[2] By the fifteenth century, both Bologna and Padua were renowned for medicine, but their law faculties were even larger. For example, in the year 1466 when Schedel obtained his doctorate in medicine, Padua awarded almost twice as many degrees in law as it did in medicine.[3]

Universities in Europe stipulated a course of study based on a set of common texts. In medicine, these were works written by (or at least attributed to) the Greek medical authors Hippocrates (*c.* 460–*c.* 370 BCE) and Galen (129–*c.* 216 CE); commentaries on these works by Arabic authors known in Europe as Johannitius (Hunayn ibn Ishaq, 809–873), Rhazes (Muhammad ibn Zakariya al-Razi, *c.* 865–*c.* 925), and Avicenna (Ibn Sina, *c.* 980–1037); and more recent European commentaries by university professors.[4] All of these texts were read and taught in Latin. The Greek texts had been translated into Latin from the Arabic versions (some of which were based on editions in Syriac) alongside their Arabic commentaries during the twelfth and thirteenth centuries. A list that Schedel made of the lectures he had attended at Padua confirms that these works were still taught in the middle of the fifteenth century:

> [In the first year,]
> Doctor Matteolo Mattioli of Perugia, king of physicians of our age, has read all the seven parts of *Aphorisms* and the book on *Prognostics* of the most ancient Hippocrates.
>   Doctor Paolo Bagellardo of Fiume has read the first fen [part] of the fourth [book] of Avicenna's *Canon* and *On Urines* by Gilles de Corbeil [*c.* 1140–*c.* 1224].
>   Doctor Francesco Noale has read the book, *Small Art of Medicine*, by Galen and the tract *On Urines* by Avicenna.
>   Doctor Matteo Boldiero of Verona has read the ninth book of Almansor [Rhazes, *Book of Medicine to Mansur*] and several fens of the third book of Avicenna's *Canon*, namely parts 10, 9, 18, 19, 21, etc.

In the second year,

Doctor Mattioli, ordinary professor of theoretical medicine, has read all four fens of the first book of Avicenna's *Canon* as well as Avicenna on the powers of the heart.

Doctor Girolamo dalle Valli, knight, has read the ninth book by Rhazes to Almansor.

Doctor Francesco Noale has read the *Aphorisms* of Hippocrates.

Doctor Matteo Boldiero of Verona, ordinary professor in practical medicine, has read the first fen of the fourth book of *Canon* with the exposition of Gentile da Foligno [d. 1348], and the second fen of [the same book] of *Canon*, and on feast days [he has read] the surgery of Avicenna, namely the third, fourth and fifth fens of the fourth book [of *Canon*].

In the third year,

Doctor Mattioli, prince of physicians, read firstly the first part of *Problems* of Aristotle with an explanation by the Conciliator [Peter of Abano, 1250–1316], and the book *Small Art of Medicine* of Galen and *Isagoge* of Johannitius.

Doctor Paolo Bagellardo of Fiume has read the first fen of the fourth book of *Canon*, on fevers.

Doctor Francesco Noale has read the first fen of the first book of *Canon* and a tract on pulses and urine by Avicenna.

Doctor Baldassarre Gemini of Perugia has read the ninth [book] of Almansor with Avicenna's introduction in the third book [of *Canon*].

I also heard [lectures on] surgery by Doctor Antonio Mussato in the first year, by Doctor Angelo in the second year, and by Dr Matheo in the third year.

In 1465, I was at the solemn celebration of an
anatomy of the human body.[5]

The list of the illustrious professors at Padua and the books
they had expounded was no doubt a reminder of the education Schedel was proud to have completed. His singling out of
Matteolo Mattioli (d. *c.* 1473) as 'king of physicians of our age' is
understandable since Mattioli was the 'ordinary professor of theoretical medicine'. Contrary to our modern sense of the adjective
'ordinary' relative to 'extraordinary', an 'ordinary' professor in
this period meant a senior professor with higher standing (and
salary) than the junior, 'extraordinary' professor. In fact, some
European universities still retain the title of 'professor ordinarius'
for their most distinguished academics. According to the standard division of medicine at the time, professors in the medical
faculty were assigned to teach either 'theory' (general principles
governing health and disease) or 'practice' (general rules relating
to particular diseases and their treatment), with practice usually
deemed the lesser of the two in standing. The 'ordinary professor
of theoretical medicine' – as Mattioli was – was therefore the
highest-ranking professor in the medical faculty.

In a three-year cycle, professors of theoretical medicine were
required to read book one (on physiology) of Avicenna's *Canon*,
the Hippocratic *Aphorisms* and *Prognostics*, and Galen's *Small Art of
Medicine*, while professors of practical medicine read the fourth
book (on fevers) of *Canon* and the ninth book (symptoms and
treatments of particular diseases) of Rhazes's *Book of Medicine to
Mansur*.[6] Though the statutes only required medical students to
have heard lectures of the ordinary professors, lectures on the
same books (offered a year after those by the ordinary professors) by the extraordinary professors must have been helpful
for revision or preparation ahead of the ordinary professor's
lectures. The frequent reference to Avicenna's *Canon* in Schedel's

list attests to its usefulness as a compilation of views of various writers within a broadly Aristotelian framework, covering a wide range of medical topics from physiology, fevers and diseases to remedies and surgery. Given the Aristotelian foundation of the arts curriculum, *Canon* rendered medical instruction coherent and continuous with concepts students had learned earlier. In particular, its first section was a well-known focal point for debating the status of medicine: whether it was demonstrative knowledge or non-demonstrative like an art or a craft, and how it related to natural philosophy.[7]

Tacked on at the end of Schedel's list of professors and their books were the names of three professors of surgery. These posts were somewhat different from the other professorships in that they were not divided into ordinary and extraordinary. The requirement for holding the post was at least four years' surgical experience, though not necessarily a medical degree.[8] There was no standard text associated with this position. It was left to the lecturer to find useful works that covered practical procedures such as bloodletting, cataract operation, cauterization of wounds or removal of fistula. These were necessary for those seeking a surgical degree, but less important for those pursuing a medical doctorate. The rather cursory form in which Schedel recorded the surgery lectures without any mention of texts may well reflect their perceived insignificance when compared to the lectures by the other professors.[9]

Schedel's list ended with a note that in 1465 he had attended a 'solemn celebration of an anatomy of a human body'. This was the annual anatomy stipulated for medical faculties since the fourteenth century, and for which there was a standard prescribed book, Mondino de' Liuzzi's *Anatomy* (illus. 6), partly based on Mondino's own dissections. The text described the principal organs and their functions in the order of dissection (roughly following the rate of putrefaction of the organs). Those in the abdominal cavity were tackled first, then those in the thoracic area, followed by those in the head. Structures covering the whole body such as muscles, blood vessels and bones were described at the end of the dissection rather briefly, since much of the body would have putrefied by then.

The Paduan statutes stipulated that one of the extraordinary professors should be appointed to read out the text of Mondino's *Anatomy*, while one of the ordinary professors (either of practice

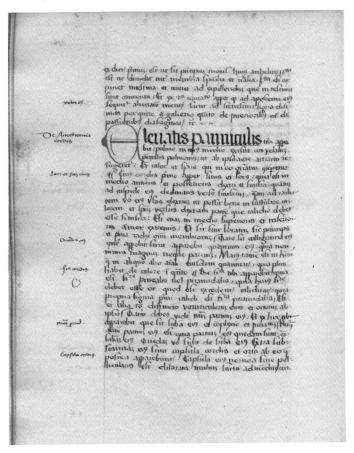

6 Schedel's copy of Mondino's *Anatomia* (not in Schedel's hand).
In the margin, a small heart-shaped sketch has been added next to
the text about the heart. Ink on paper, height 23.2 centimetres/9¹⁄₁₀ in.

or of theory) should explain the text line by line, and point out what he had explained in the text 'by visual testimony [*oculata fide*] and verify [*verificet*] it in the cadaver itself'.[10] In other words, the conduct of the annual anatomy was set out like an academic lecture of reciting a text and explaining the meaning of that text, with the addition of visual confirmation of the meaning of the text from the body. The reading and the exposition of the text were done by the extraordinary and ordinary professors respectively. The role of the professor of surgery was limited to dissecting the body, which could also be delegated to a more suitable person. The academic hierarchy was thus reflected in the annual anatomy: the ordinary professor, *not* the professor of surgery, exercised the right and authority to expound on the structure of the human body as described in a set text.

At the end of his copy of Mondino's *Anatomy*, Schedel recorded that the public anatomy at Padua was held from 20 to 24 March in the presence of all the professors and the son of the podestà of Padua.[11] It was an event where 'the smallest of doubts about the human body arising from the anatomy had all been explained away by the professors,' though he did not record what exactly had been discussed. Anatomical knowledge was undeniably important for surgery or understanding ailments, but the annual anatomy was not a supplementary lesson for any specific course of lectures. It was an institutional gathering that more resembled an academic disputation with questions and answers.[12] Professors displayed their expert, text-based knowledge on human anatomy to the academic community at large. Schedel's description of the anatomy as a 'solemn celebration' captures the sense of occasion, as professors and students came together to celebrate collectively their academic, bookish knowledge of the human body. The cadaver, Schedel noted, was buried with 'great pomp'.

Though not recorded in Schedel's list, students at Padua were also required to accompany a renowned physician on his visits to the sick for at least a year.[13] We do not know with whom Schedel had trained, but almost all the professors of medicine at Padua had a private practice. This aspect of bedside training generated a genre of writing called *consilia*, or advice on individual cases and treatments, including medicinal recipes for specific ailments. These recipes, often unique to a particular physician, were much sought after by students. Schedel collected many such *consilia* and recipes written by the professors at Padua.[14] In his Paduan notebook, on the reverse of the page listing medicinal recipes and prayers for the plague, Schedel pasted in an image of St Sebastian (illus. 7), a saint frequently invoked against the plague.[15] In this period, images of saints were believed to have the effect of warding off diseases, which explains its inclusion in a collection of recipes. The amount of time required for attending bedside visits was comparatively shorter (one year) than the time students spent learning from books (three years), but it was certainly an aspect of teaching that attracted foreign students.[16]

By the middle of the fifteenth century, students spent much of the three years of their medical course hearing lectures on a set of authoritative medical texts, amassing textual knowledge, learning how to resolve seeming contradictions or disagreements among textual authorities, and honing their own argumentative skills that they learned through lectures and debating exercises. The mode of examination was by disputation, an oral examination in front of the professors in which a candidate demonstrated his mastery of the authoritative texts.[17] In April 1466, Schedel obtained his doctorate in medicine.[18] The degree ceremony would have included a ritual of receiving a closed book which was then opened, symbolizing the knowledge the candidate had mastered and was now qualified to teach.[19] It endorsed the centrality of the book for academic knowledge.

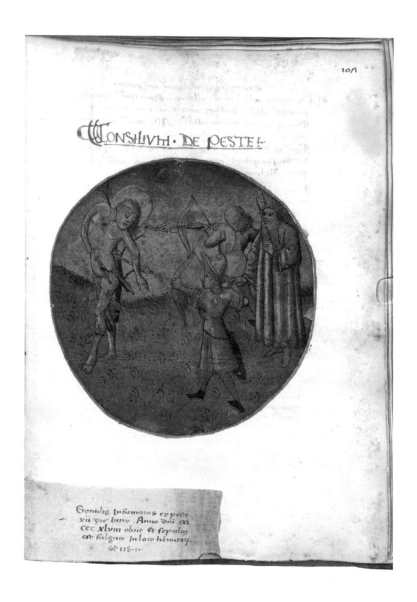

7 Drawing of the martyrdom of St Sebastian inserted into a collection of hand-written recipes that Schedel had gathered while he was in Padua, and included in the same volume as his copy of *Anatomia* (illus. 6).

SCHEDEL AND HIS BOOKS

Schedel attended Padua when the new technology of printing
with moveable type was not yet widely available in Italy. His university books were handwritten on paper or on parchment. Texts
prescribed for study had been copied by hand from another
manuscript for centuries, and since the curriculum was fairly static,
it was possible to use old copies, which Schedel's elder cousin
Hermann acquired and sent to Italy.[20] For instance, Schedel's copy
of the *Articella*, a collection of set texts of the medical curriculum,
had been compiled in the fourteenth century (illus. 8).[21] It is typical of an academic manuscript, larger in size than his *Anatomia* of
Mondino, written in double columns in a script that was angular
and woven together with numerous abbreviations characteristic
of writing that is now called 'Gothic'.[22] The visual layout helped
demarcate the words of different authorities. For example, in
Galen's commentary on Hippocrates' *Aphorisms* (one of the texts
included in the *Articella*), Hippocrates' words were written in
larger script with wider spacing between the lines than the text
of Galen's commentary. Students could insert between the lines
their professors' points on the wording of the Hippocratic text,
while those on Galen's commentary or other points were inserted
in the margins of the page. Such a layout was a familiar feature
of academic manuscripts that demarcated visually the different
authorities on the page, which also enabled structured note-taking
by students.

Schedel's manuscripts from his time at Padua indicate that
he was also studying more than what was formally required for
a medical degree. He learned ancient Greek from Demetrius
Chalcondyles, the first professor of Greek at Padua; he studied
the works of Cicero, Ovid and Horace; he copied out orations
by recent humanists such as Poggio Bracciolini, Leonardo Bruni
and Francesco Filelfo; he recorded ancient inscriptions and
ruins in Padua, Venice and Treviso; and he copied out drawings

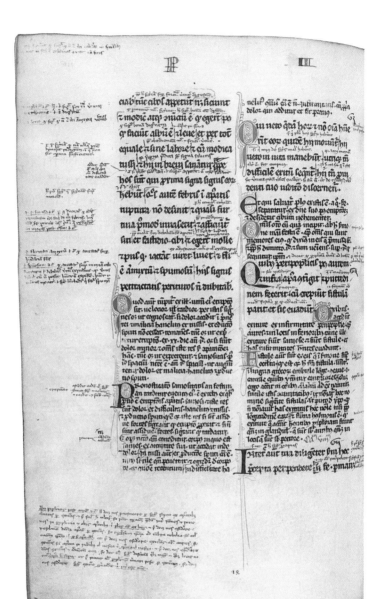

8 Schedel's copy of Galen's commentary on Hippocrates' *Aphorisms* (part of the *Articella*), on parchment, height 34.5 centimetres/13⅗ in.

and inscriptions on ancient Greek monuments recorded by Cyriaco of Ancona (1391–1452), who had spent some time with the Bishop of Padua, Pietro Donato.[23] Donato was one of the patrons who made Padua an important centre of antiquarian studies and humanist manuscript production.[24]

The Paduan scribe and illuminator Bartolomeo Sanvito as well as the painter Andrea Mantegna designed majuscules (capital letters) to achieve a 'classical' look of the inscriptions on classical monuments.[25] These were incorporated into manuscripts by humanists who adopted lettering found in older manuscripts (from

9 Example of humanist 'ancient script'. Virgil's *Aenid,* compiled in Padua, 1463, written by Franciscus de Camuciis, with the last five lines in capital letters by Bartolomeo Sanvito. On parchment, height 23.8 centimetres/9⅜ in.

the eleventh or twelfth centuries rather than from the ancient period) of classical texts for minuscules (lower-case letters).[26] This 'ancient script' (littera antiqua) was written with round, upright, well-spaced letters with fewer abbreviations in a single column (illus. 9).

Schedel learned at Padua that works of humanists and classical authors had a distinctive appearance on the page, different from the closely woven Gothic script arranged in double columns of his medical texts (illus. 8). His growing sensitivity towards the visual dimension of lettering may be detected in his interest in letter forms and the fact that he changed his handwriting to incorporate some features of humanist lettering.[27]

When Schedel left Padua and began practising medicine, first in Nördlingen and then at his home town, Nuremberg, he did not leave behind the world of books.[28] Printing was a new technology that replicated manuscripts swiftly, and early printers preserved the look of manuscripts by using different type fonts.[29] The Venetian printer Nicolas Jenson, who was acquainted with Paduan scribes such as Sanvito, printed books of classical authors with the type now known as 'roman', modelled on the 'ancient script' of humanist manuscripts. He also printed large academic books with 'Gothic' type in double columns recognizable to Schedel's generation of university students as similar in appearance to their manuscript texts.[30] Schedel bought printed books of both kinds. Acquiring printed books did not induce him to throw away his earlier manuscripts, however. He continued to revisit his manuscripts and notes from his student days and augmented them with additional notes from printed books, while he also inserted handwritten notes and indexes into his printed books. Both manuscripts and printed books were adorned with additional drawings and printed images framed with coloured ink. This was by no means unusual at the time, and it may also be a habit that he picked up while in Padua (illus. 7).[31] There was

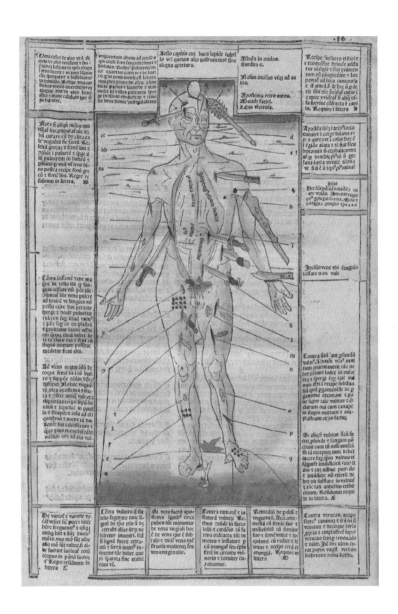

10 *A Little Collection of Medicine* (1495), 'wound man', from Schedel's copy.
Page height 43 centimeters/17 in.

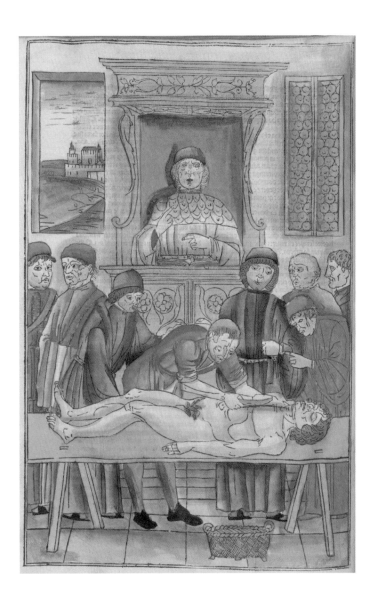

11 *A Little Collection of Medicine* (1495), dissection scene, from Schedel's copy.

no distinction between printed and handwritten books for Schedel – he cherished and adorned them alike.

Schedel notwithstanding, the market for printed medical books seems not to have been as large or reliable as that for law books in this period.[32] What appears to have been a modest commercial success was a slender volume of eighty large pages with woodcut illustrations, *A Little Collection of Medicine* (*Fasciculus medicinae*), printed six times by the Venetian printers Giovanni and Gregorio de Gregoriis, and fourteen more times by others to 1530.[33] Schedel had a copy of the 1495 edition. This book was a compilation of short practical texts on uroscopy, the astrological connections of parts of the human body, bloodletting points, types of wounds, diseases and their remedies. The image of a naked man assailed by various weapons (illus. 10) succinctly summarized the external injuries the human body could sustain. The figure hints at a pose that art historians call 'contrapposto' where the weight of the body is placed on one leg, with the other leg balanced towards the back, causing the torso to twist slightly. It is a pose that was adopted in later anatomical works, including *Fabrica*.

A Little Collection of Medicine included (from the 1493 edition) the text of Mondino's *Anatomy* with a full-page woodcut (illus. 11). It shows a figure reading the text at the top centre, below whom is another figure to the right leaning over the cadaver and pointing. At the centre is a barber with a knife about to cut open the cadaver. He is flanked by two younger figures and there are older men standing at the back. As the historian Jerome Bylebyl pointed out, this woodcut is a fair representation of a public anatomy as specified in the Paduan statutes, set down around the time that Schedel was studying.[34] Though the content of *A Little Collection* printed thirty years after his student days was hardly new to Schedel, he may well have appreciated this woodcut scene as a reminder of his time at Padua. It is also likely that Vesalius had this image in mind when he caricatured the contemporary practice of

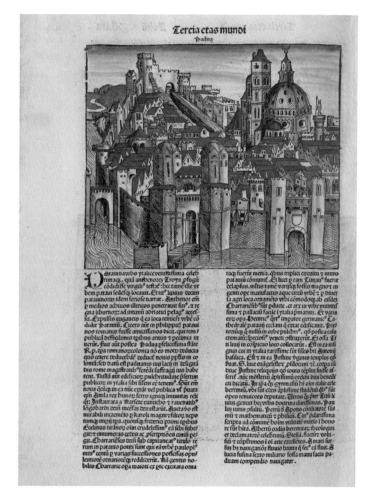

anatomy in the preface to *Fabrica* – those 'aloft in their chairs' croaking away 'like jackdaws', and those performing the actual dissection who 'hacked things up for display' with no under-standing of what it was that they were dissecting.[35]

Schedel formed a library that was learned, large and respect-able, stocked with manuscripts and printed books on academic

12 The city of Padua. Schedel's own, hand-coloured copy of *The Book of Chronicles* (1493). Page height *c.* 47 centimetres/18½ in.

and humanist topics. It contained material that was of interest
to his neighbours in Nuremberg. One of them, Albrecht Dürer,
was inspired to draw some mythical figures based on drawings
in Cyriaco's manuscript Schedel had copied at Padua.[36] Another
was the university-educated merchant and patron of humanist
scholars and artists Sebald Schreyer.[37] Schreyer spearheaded and
financed with his brother-in-law a large, illustrated publication
on the history of the world and Nuremberg's place in it. *The Book
of Chronicles* (now commonly known as the *Nuremberg Chronicle*)
was printed in 1493. Schedel provided the text compiled from his
own notes on inscriptions and antiquities from his time in Italy
as well as other books and manuscripts in his library.[38] The artists
Michael Wolgemut and Wilhelm Pleydenwurff were contracted
to design the woodcuts. The printer Anton Koberger commissioned a smaller size of type to preserve the original layout.
Although he had recently printed the Roman poet Virgil's works
in roman type (1492), Koberger opted for Gothic type, which he
had been using for most of the Latin works he had printed. *The
Book of Chronicles* was illustrated extensively, which was achieved by
reusing woodcuts – for example the cityscape for Padua (illus. 12)
stood in for Marseille, Metz and Nicea also, but each of them was
coloured differently, rendering them visually distinct.[39] This was
a way to economize on woodcuts while also making them relevant to a specific city. Schedel was no stranger to using colour in
books to individualize them. His own copy of *The Book of Chronicles*
was further personalized with additional images, decorations
and annotations.

　　Becoming a university-educated physician meant becoming
immersed in a world of books. Schedel's experience is a helpful
example of how this was achieved. At Padua, he learned through
books – by hearing lectures about them, making copies of them,
annotating them, and mastering them for disputations. In extending his intellectual horizons with the more recent developments

of humanist scholarship, he became sensitized to the different look of manuscripts, developed an interest in letter forms and changed his handwriting. He continued to collect books after getting his medical degree. While he did not publish a book on medicine, the historical material he began gathering in Padua became the basis of *The Book of Chronicles*.

For Schedel, books – whether handwritten or printed – were not just conveyors of abstract ideas or collectable objects to be preserved in mint condition. He added to them notes and indexes for his own use, inserted illuminations, glued in prints and drawings, and added coloured frames and rubrics to create a visual experience that was unique to him. Books were the material support and expression of a learned world, and Schedel engaged with them actively, personally and visually. He was proud of his library as a mark of learning and respectability that should be preserved by his family and descendants.

Schedel was a transitional figure in straddling the medieval curriculum of medical study and humanist interest in the textual and material remains of the classical world, and he embraced both handwritten and printed books. His own foray into the world of publication was on universal history, not on medicine. His *Book of Chronicles* may well have helped cement his reputation as a learned figure among the Nuremberg elite, which in turn may have benefited what was an already successful medical career. He did not, however, write books about medicine in order to further his career or demonstrate his intellectual credentials. These were possibilities pursued by others.

TWO

Books and Careers

y the turn of the sixteenth century the printed book was here to stay, despite the financial and practical challenges of getting published, as its intellectual and social potential began to be recognized.[1] Anatomy, though occupying a marginal status in academic medicine, became a topic on which university-educated physicians began to publish books well before Vesalius came on the scene. I discuss a selection of examples in this chapter that demonstrates how learned authors sought to elevate their subject by seeking endorsement of the social elite, and update it with the latest humanist scholarship and personal insights. They believed that printed books could help build their authority and advance their careers. Vesalius would learn much from these books.

HUMANIST SCHOLARS AND ANATOMY

Aldus Manutius (c. 1451–1515) was a scholar who established a printing business in Venice in the 1490s to promote humanist learning and scholarship. He was supported in this venture by a nobleman-philosopher, Giovanni Pico of Mirandola, and his nephew Alberto Pio, prince of Carpi (about 20 kilometres/ 12 mi. southwest of Mirandola). Aldus had met Giovanni Pico at the University of Ferrara, a centre for the study of ancient Greek that produced scholars such as Niccolò Leoniceno, who advocated the need to consult ancient Greek medical authors in order to correct the errors of subsequent writers such as Pliny the Elder or Avicenna. On Pico's recommendation, Aldus became tutor to Giovanni's nephews Alberto and Leonello at Carpi.[2]

Aldus began printing with a book on Greek grammar so that more could learn to read the works he went on to publish, such as those by Aristophanes, Homer and others. Greek fonts were commissioned, designed and cast for these books. The books

13 The Greek text of *On Anatomical Procedures*, in Galen's *Works* by the Aldine firm (1525), with every ten lines numbered in the outer margin. Page height 32.7 centimetres/12⅞ in.

were dedicated to men distinguished by rank or learning or both.
Aldus likened them to 'shields' that protected his work, which
would in turn carry 'more weight' with readers.[3] In the preface
to the complete works of Aristotle (printed 1495–8), Aldus
expressed his hope to Alberto Pio of publishing all the works of
Galen in Greek.[4] But these did not see the light of day until ten
years after Aldus's own death, mainly because of the sheer amount
of the material involved, which in the end totalled more than
2,900 scholarly pages in five hefty volumes. It included, though
incomplete, Galen's *On Anatomical Procedures*, presumed to have
been lost for a long time (illus. 13).[5]

The large, hefty books such as the complete works of Galen
were meant for the bookshelf at home. Aldus then introduced a
new look to classical texts by printing them in a smaller size (half
the page height of Galen's works) with type based on a slanted
cursive hand used by earlier humanists for swifter writing, now
known as italics. As he wrote in his dedication to Marino Sanudo
– a Venetian patrician with a keen interest in humanist scholarship – these portable books of classical authors were for the busy
elite like Sanudo to take with them on their daily business.[6] The
Greek, roman and italic types that visibly marked out humanist
books gradually became features of learned medical books as more
university-educated physicians took note of humanist scholarship. Like Aldus, they also saw dedications as an opportunity to
promote their own work.

When Alessandro Benedetti (1452–1512), an acquaintance
of Aldus, published *A Description of the Human Body or On Anatomical
Matters* (*Historia corporis humani sive anatomice*) in 1502, his humanist
orientation was visible in several ways. The last word in the Latin
title, 'anatomice', was a transliteration of the Greek adjective
'anatomical', and signalled the author's interest in the Greek
language. The text was printed in roman type in a single column,
and decorative initials were used at the start of each chapter. Some

of the initials were faceted in imitation of classical inscriptions (illus. 14).

Benedetti was born in Verona and studied at Padua, where he met other humanist scholars, including some Venetian patricians.[7] He spent several years as a physician visiting various Venetian territories including Greece and Crete, which gave him an opportunity to collect Greek manuscripts. He then settled in Venice, joined the College of Physicians, and began practising there. Though physicians were excluded from political office in Venice, they had been mixing socially and culturally with the ruling elite through their common interest in literature and learning.[8] Books could play a part in developing cultural ties with the Venetian elite.

Benedetti began publishing slender, medium-sized books (page height *c.* 20 centimetres/7⅞ in.) in Latin on medical topics – on medical aphorisms (1493) dedicated to Sanudo, and on pestilence (1493) addressed to a Venetian senator Giacomo Contarini. After serving in the Venetian campaign against Charles VIII of France, Benedetti published in 1496 his experience in *A Diary of the Caroline War*, recording the cases he had treated alongside some harrowing details of a battle and a siege. It was printed by Aldus and dedicated to the rulers of Venice, namely the Doge and members of the Council of Ten. Though written in Italian probably because it was of interest to a wider audience, this work was nevertheless a humanist project in spirit – to preserve for posterity the triumph of the Venetians just as ancient historians like Thucydides and Livy had written first-hand accounts of war.

A Description of the Human Body (1502) was also medium sized (150 pages, page height *c.* 21 centimetres/8¼ in.). It was dedicated to the Holy Roman Emperor Maximilian I – an erstwhile ally of the Venetian Republic. Citing classical rulers such as Alexander the Great as precedents, Benedetti praised Maximilian for his learning and interest in understanding the workings of nature.

ri folent uàna pquírēteſ/cerebrūm pforatum putauit:co
gnito a phyſico errore:ſpecillū inter geminatas utraſq̃
membranas impoſuiſſe cognouit.

De cauis cerebri.   Cap. x.

Vnt & in cerebro terni ſpecus prioris gemi
ní ſunt tenuiſſima irus círcūdāte mēbrana.
Poſtremi uero cauum p ſe ſine membrana
conſiſtit/ſed ſua dūtaxat duricia oſeruat͛/iſ
li gemini cōſtituti ſunt/ſicut & pleraq̃ mē
bra: renes: pulmōes:aures oculi:ut ſi qd alteri pti occur
rat:reliqua illæſa ſuo fungat͛ numere:in cerebro.n.uita
lis ſpūs:q a corde ſurſum uerſus arteriis diffundit͛:tēpe
rat͛/atq̃ ſenſificā inde uirtute/quā aíalē uocant/recipit.
quæ ex iis cauernis ſpūs ipſos q & ſpiramēta uocantur/
ſenſib9neruis:muſculiſq̃ motus ac uarias potēias p mē
bra diffuſas adminiſtrāt:q̃ ſi uertígine ſpōtanea aut:p uí
circuagēdo corp9equo uel nauícuā uel morbo:ut i uer
tiginoſis turbata ſūt/humores & ſpūs ſimul exagitēt/uñ
functiōibus ſuis deſtituis:audit9uiſus:motuſq̃ mēbro
rū cū uniuerſo corpore in ruinā plabat͛/cerebri materia
paulatim ſeccāda eſt:quoad internæ appareāt cauernæ
quæ uiuētibus ampliores ſunt:in dextra.ſ.& ſiniſtra par
te/utraq̃.n.eiuſdē rōnis eſt:ambígunt tm̄ philoſophā
tes an geminas imagines ſiue ſpēs(Cicero ſpectra uo
cat)referat uterq̃ ſinus/ cū loco differant neq̃ in aliquo
tertio conueníant:ut oculis contingit: qui & ſi gemini
ſint unicam tamen repræſentent formā:In his enim ſen
ſuum nobiliſſimorum uires habentur/ex his cogitatio
nis:exſtimationiſq̃ atq̃ intellectus potentia adipiſcitur/
in his qui communis ſenſus dicitur ſubiectorum ſenſibi

He was careful to call anatomy a branch of philosophy, distancing the emperor from the actual business of dissection ('leaving
to surgeons and physicians the distasteful task of cutting'), and
emphasized the contemplation of divine creation as behoving
an emperor.[9]

Benedetti set the scene of his book as a public anatomy, which
was made all the more convincing by including some details of
how to arrange one: the cadaver of a hanged ignoble who could

14 Roman type and a faceted initial in Benedetti, *Anatomice* (1502).
Page height *c.* 21 centimetres/8¼ in.

not be recognized locally should be used; the executed person should be middle-aged, not too thin or fat, but tall enough for the audience to be able to see; a temporary semicircular structure like the ancient theatres in Verona (his home town) or Rome should be erected; and two treasurers should be chosen to collect fees to buy the necessary equipment such as razors, knives, hooks and sponges.[10] Benedetti's scholarly friends and patricians were invited to join Maximilian at the theatre.[11] This was a fictional gathering rather than a record of what had actually taken place. Yet these were Benedetti's true audience. The distinguished guests were described as attending at night after they had concluded their own business of the day, and stayed long after the medical students had left, to contemplate the human body. It was the support of the emperor and the learned elite that ennobled the study of anatomy.

Benedetti hoped to improve the description (in Latin) of the human body because there were too many 'barbaric' and erroneous words derived from the Arabic.[12] He suggested the use of 'omentum' (meaning apron in Latin) instead of the Arabic 'zirbus', and 'siphac' was replaced by 'peritoneum', derived from the Greek. Some Greek anatomical terms were transliterated, such as 'choledochus' (gall bladder) and 'opisthenar' (back of the hand). Ailments and treatments too had Greek names: a tumour in the groin was 'bubonocoele', and 'paracentesis' indicated a procedure puncturing the abdomen to draw liquid in cases of dropsy. Benedetti cited his patrician friend Pietro Bembo, who could read better in the dark than in daylight, as an example of the condition 'nyctalopes' (the modern meaning of 'nyctalopia' for anglophones is an inability to see in poor light, rather than night vision as is the case in French, but both meanings were present in classical texts).[13] Benedetti thus 'hellenized' the words with which to describe the human body and its ailments and treatments. To these were added unusual cases he had encountered – for instance, a Greek man in Crete sneezed out a steel arrowhead by which he had been wounded twenty years earlier. Benedetti ended the book by urging physicians and surgeons to attend annual dissections in a theatre, for the contemplation of the work of nature revealed therein.

Benedetti, a humanist physician with proficiency in Greek and practising in Venice, was thus promoting himself among the Venetian elites through publications, among which was his medium-sized book on anatomy dedicated to Maximilian. Though it did not lead to any imperial favour, it certainly consolidated Benedetti's reputation in Venice, where he was reasonably well off by the time of his death in 1512.[14] It was a precedent that emboldened Vesalius to dedicate his book to Maximilian's grandson Charles V.

JACOPO BERENGARIO – MASTER SURGEON

Another acquaintance of Aldus was Jacopo Berengario of Carpi (1460–1530), the son of a surgeon in Carpi who served the Pio family.[15] Berengario likely met Aldus when Aldus was tutoring Alberto Pio. Berengario trained with his father and obtained a degree in arts and medicine from Bologna in 1489. He then spent some time in Rome where his connection with the Pio family may have opened doors for him. He retained his wealthy clients when he returned to Bologna to teach surgery in 1502, the same year Benedetti published his book on anatomy. In contrast to Benedetti, Berengario foregrounded his surgical expertise, though he too aimed high in his dedications.

In 1518, Berengario treated a skull injury sustained by the Lord of Florence, Lorenzo II de' Medici (1492–1519). He promptly advertised his success in a book (210 pages, page height *c.* 21 centimetres/8¼ in.), *A Very Useful and Complete Tract on the Fracture of the Skull*, dedicated to his noble patient, though Lorenzo died

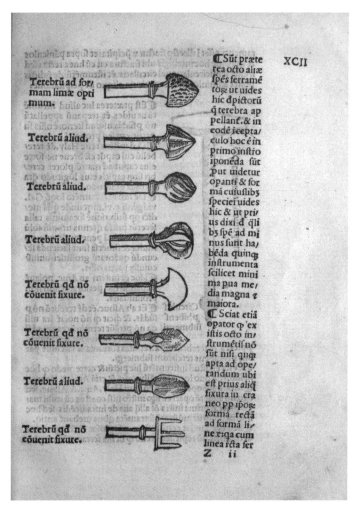

soon afterwards. In this book, Berengario demonstrated how his
knowledge of treating skull injuries was consistent with the views
of medical authorities such as Avicenna, Albucasis (Al-Zahrawi),
Haly Abbas (Ali ibn al Abbas al-Majusi) or Galen. He explained
the shape and use of the instruments discussed by these authors

15 'The prudent physician always has ready his instruments of all shapes
and many in number.' Berengario, *On the Fracture of the Skull* (1518).
Page height *c.* 21 centimetres/8¼ in.

and illustrated the need to use a drill bit that matched the specific shape of the injury when trepanning the skull (illus. 15). In his view, a 'prudent physician' should always have to hand many different types of instruments and, where necessary, have one made to treat a specific injury, even if it ended up being used only once.[16] A cabinet full of instruments was a sign of a responsible physician, since an instrument ill-suited to a purpose would mean that the physician would have nothing but his 'uncertain hand' to guide it and could put a patient's life at risk.[17] Instruments designed for specific injuries were thus a mark of expertise and reliability for Berengario, the professor of surgery.

Berengario went on to publish a commentary on Mondino's *Anatomy* in 1521.[18] The title page showed an architectural frame with ornate columns (illus. 16) flanking the title of the book (printed in red). The coat of arms and the name of Pope Leo X (1475–1521) were shown at the top, and the base of the left column bore the coat of arms of the Pio family. The book was dedicated to Leo's cousin Giulio de' Medici (1478–1534), soon to be Pope Clement VII, who had briefly been Bishop of Bologna in 1518. At the bottom of the title page is a dissection scene with a seated professor, a dissector at the table and three spectators. At this point Berengario was over fifty years old, and already had an established reputation with clients in high places – in his book, he mentioned his acquaintance with the Medici family as well as the powerful Bentivoglio family of Bologna.[19] This publication was meant to cement his status in academia. As professor of surgery, he was claiming the authority to comment on Mondino's text, a role usually reserved for his more senior, distinguished colleagues.

Berengario's commentary (page height *c.* 21 centimetres/ 8¼ in.) used the same size of paper as his surgical tract but ran to more than a thousand pages, printed in roman type in a single column. Despite the appearance of his book, Berengario's approach to humanist scholarship was tempered by his own training as a

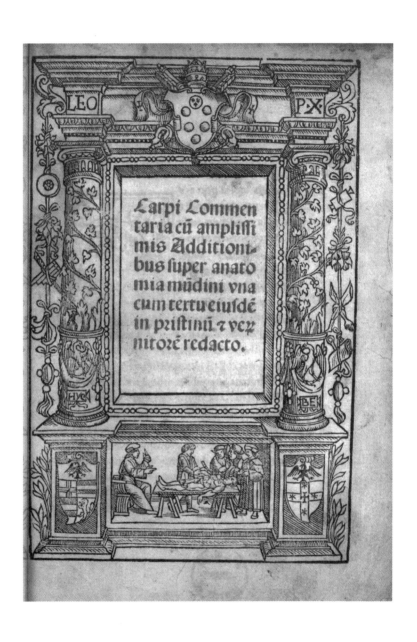

16 Berengario's *Commentary on Mondino's Anatomy* (1521), title page. Page height *c.* 21 centimetres/8¼ in.

surgeon. He acknowledged humanist efforts to establish medical terminology based on Greek terms, but was critical of discarding Arabic terminology altogether. For example, Leoniceno translated the Greek 'peritoneon' into Latin as an 'interior abdominal membrane' in order to avoid using the word 'siphac', but the alternative description made it difficult to understand Galen's comments on it.[20] Terminological confusion could also lead to surgical errors. In criticizing humanist scholars, Berengario invoked a well-known phrase indicating the limits of human authority: 'Plato is my friend, but truth is my greater friend.'[21]

According to Berengario, a good anatomist ought to know not just the works of ancients such as Aristotle or Galen, but also the writings of Avicenna and more recent authors.[22] Among recent authors, Mondino – Berengario's distinguished predecessor at Bologna – was singled out for his 'divine genius' because he had written a succinct manual on dissection, especially in the absence (as Berengario then believed) of Galen's *On Anatomical Procedures*. Berengario identified with Mondino, and saw himself as similarly engaged in the use of hands (*operatio manualis*) – as he frequently wrote: '*I* have anatomized' (*ego anatomizavi*). He proudly related his own dissection of a pregnant woman in a public anatomy attended by 'almost five hundred students and citizens'. Public anatomies (Berengario called them 'common anatomies') using a single body were, however, of limited value since some structures had to be destroyed in order to reach others. Instead, he advocated frequent private dissections of humans as well as animals. This book was thus a professor of surgery's defence of anatomy that emphasized the work of the hand as the foundation of anatomical knowledge.

Berengario argued that the determination of the existence and shape of an organ belonged to dissection using the senses of sight and touch. This was called 'anatomy of the senses' (*anatomia sensibilis*) and Berengario believed that the senses were sufficient to contradict the words of others.[23] The best-known example of this approach was the rejection of 'the wondrous net' (*rete mirabile*) of arteries described by Galen as situated underneath the base of the brain inside the skull. The *rete mirabile* exists in some animals, but not in humans. Even after anatomizing 'more than a hundred times', Berengario could not find it. He then inserted a thin stylus through the carotid arteries in the brain which reached the skull without resistance. If the arteries were entangled into a net, there should have been resistance. There was none. Berengario therefore concluded that Galen must have imagined this structure, and others after him had simply taken his word for it.[24] An instrument thus helped confirm Berengario's discovery.

The emphasis on the work of the hands meant that the practitioner of the 'anatomy of the senses' was a 'master craftsman of the senses' (*artifex sensibilis*). This type of anatomy was elevated by Berengario, who described God himself as *the* master craftsman (*primus artifex*).[25] Knowledge derived from dissections could correct terminological confusion of the humanists and morphological errors of others. Aware of the problem of trust when he criticized other authorities in his dissections, he stated that he had dissected more than a hundred times, and that testimony of multiple witnesses would be helpful.[26]

The *Commentary* included many tips for surgical procedures, some of which were illustrated by woodcuts. At the end of the book, Berengario included images of structures that were often discussed only cursorily at the end of an actual anatomy. These included muscles of the whole body, which were shown in the round from three angles – the front, the back and the side. These figures not only helped physicians improve their prognosis and surgical knowledge (illus. 17), but could also teach painters how to draw human muscles.[27] Understanding the arrangement of abdominal muscles enabled expert painters to depict the skin following the contours of the underlying muscles, for example.[28]

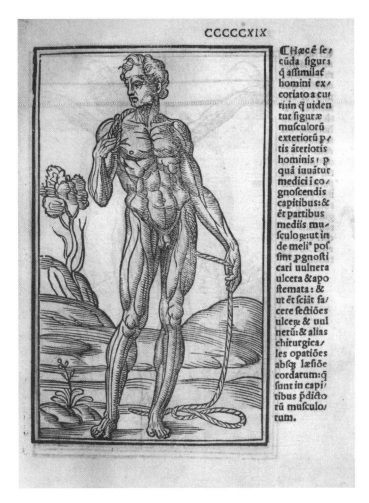

CCCCCXIX

℘Hæcê se
cúda figura
q̃ aſſimilat
homini ex
coriato a cui
ti:in q̃ uiden
tut figuræ
muſculorū
exteriorū p
tis ātetiotis
hominis (p
quā iuuátut
medici i co
gnoſcendis
capitibus:&
ēt partibus
mediis mu
ſculo℞:ut in
de meli° poſ
ſint ℘gnoſti
cari uulnera
ulcera &apo
ſtemata: &
ut ēt ſciāt fa
cere ſectiōes
ulce℞ & uul
netū:& alias
chirurgica
les opatiōes
abſq̃ læſiōe
cordarum:q̃
ſunt in capi
tibus p̃dicto
rū muſculo
rum.

We do not know for certain who the craftsmen were, but it is likely that Berengario oversaw the production of the images that made reference to artistic themes.[29] The muscle figure with the noose (illus. 17) is reminiscent of Michelangelo's David, and the posterior view of the skeleton holding two skulls (illus. 18) includes an open stone tomb often featured in paintings of

17 'By this picture physicians . . . may better prognosticate wounds, ulcers and abscesses, and know how to make . . . other surgical operations without damaging the tendons.' Berengario, *Commentary* (1520).

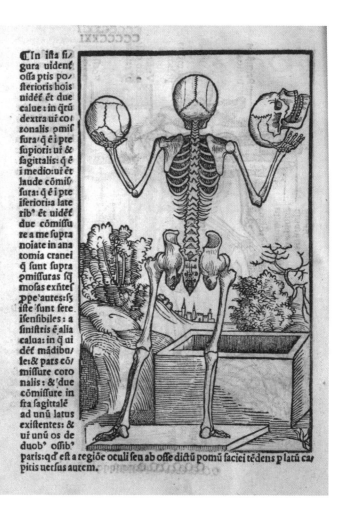

Christ's resurrection. These reflect Berengario's interest in art – his collection included a marble torso, a painting attributed to Raphael and a silver jug by Benevenuto Cellini.[30] Invoking artistic themes in his woodcuts was likely a way to signal his taste for fine art that he shared with his noble clients and to dignify the anatomized body.

18 Skeleton from the back in front of an open tomb, with two additional skulls shown from different angles. Berengario, *Commentary* (1520).

A year after his commentary on Mondino's *Anatomy*, Berengario produced another book, *A Short, Pellucid and Very Profitable Introduction to the Anatomy of the Human Body*. The pages were the same size (page height *c.* 21 centimetres/8¼ in.) as the commentary, but the book was indeed much shorter (144 pages), as promised in the title. Several woodcuts from the commentary were reused.[31] This *Introduction* omitted the polemical arguments against others, and focused on brief descriptions and functions of organs, retaining Mondino's order of dissection and terminology, with the addition of some equivalent words in Greek. The book was dedicated to Alberto Pio, with whom (Berengario reminded the dedicatee) he was taught by Aldus.[32] If Berengario had hoped for an appointment in Alberto's court, it was not to be, as Carpi fell to the imperial forces of Charles V in 1525. Berengario was called briefly to Rome by Pope Clement VII (the dedicatee of his *Commentary*) at the end of 1525 and the beginning of 1526. By 1529, he had become surgeon to Alfonso I d'Este (1499–1534), Duke of Ferrara, who now ruled Carpi.

Berengario's last publication in 1529 was an edition of Galen's anatomical works, and included the first printing in Latin of Galen's *On Anatomical Procedures*. Demetrius Chalcondyles, Schedel's teacher, had access to a Greek manuscript from which he had made a Latin translation.[33] A humanist scholar and tutor to the Gonzaga family, Lazarro Bonamico, drew Berengario's attention to Chalcondyles's translation sometime after the publication of his *Introduction* (1522).[34] *On Anatomical Procedures* was an important work that indicated Galen had advocated first-hand dissection, but in an order different from Mondino's. Galen likened the bones to the walls of a house (Galen's father was an architect) that defined features of other parts of the body.[35] The study of anatomy should therefore start with the bones and other structures common to the entire body such as muscles, veins, arteries and nerves. Galen then proposed to proceed to the alimentary and respiratory organs, the brain and the organs for reproduction (as he had done in *On the Usefulness of the Parts*), though the last part from the brain onwards was no longer extant in the Greek manuscripts.

Berengario's edition was dedicated to Ercole Gonzaga (1505–1563), son of the Marquess of Mantua and now a cardinal, who had attended the University of Bologna. In the preface, Berengario recalled the particular favour Ercole had shown him at Bologna by inviting him to a dinner with Ercole's tutor Bonamico, the famed professor of philosophy Pietro Pomponazzi and other academics.[36] Berengario had mentioned at the dinner that he had been correcting Chalcondyles's translation which Ercole then encouraged him to publish. The extent of Berengario's actual contribution to this edition is unclear, as Bonamico also appears to have been involved. It was published with Berengario named as the sole editor, however. He never missed a chance to draw the noble elite's attention to his attainments by means of books, as it was a way to maintain and consolidate his reputation.

Berengario's books are the most significant precedent for Vesalius, though Vesalius never mentioned him. It is unlikely he did not know of Berengario's work, since Bernardino Vitali, who reprinted Berengario's *Introduction* in 1535, would print Vesalius's anatomical sheets three years later. Berengario had the idea of producing two books on anatomy with shared illustrations: one thick and learned, the other thin and concise. Vesalius produced *Fabrica* and *Epitome*.[37] Berengario acknowledged that images could be useful for physicians as well as painters. So did Vesalius. Showing the body in the round from three angles set against a landscape and figures reminiscent of famous sculptures was a pictorial feature that was copied and surpassed by *Fabrica*'s woodcuts. A major difference was the size of the books.

1536 – DRYANDER AND MASSA

By the 1530s, publications in academic medicine were routinely printed in roman type. In 1536, two more books on anatomy appeared that were important to Vesalius: *Anatomy of the Head* by Johannes Dryander (1500–1560) and *An Introductory Book of Anatomy* by Niccolò Massa (d. 1569). For them, their anatomical books were among several other works they had published.

Johannes Dryander developed an interest in medicine and mathematics when young – he worked with the humanist physician Euricius Cordus, and the town clerk, surveyor, practical mathematician and instrument maker Jakob Köbel. Dryander studied at the universities of Erfurt, Bourges and Paris. At Paris he studied mathematics with Oronce Finé and medicine with Jacques Dubois.[38] He also provided illustrations for the Parisian edition of Albrecht Dürer's book on geometry and measurement.[39] It is possible that Dryander met Vesalius at Paris. At some point, Dryander was in correspondence with Vesalius, though he felt that he had not been given the respect he deserved in *Fabrica*.[40]

In 1535, Dryander was appointed ordinary professor of medicine at the University of Marburg and conducted two public anatomies in June 1535 and March 1536.[41] In September 1536, *Anatomy of the Head* was published, comprising eleven woodcuts of sequential stages of the dissection of the brain, with four or five structures labelled in each image and their names printed on the opposite page facing the woodcut. The drawings were done by Dryander and the woodcuts are attributed to Georg Thomas of Basle. It was a short tract (page height *c.* 20 centimetres/7⅞ in.) comprising 28 pages printed in roman type. Some of the woodcuts were accompanied by instruments such as a sharp knife, an 'orbicular saw' (illus. 19), pincers or forked prongs, indicating Dryander's parallel interest in instruments. These drew attention to the skill involved in dissecting the brain. In the

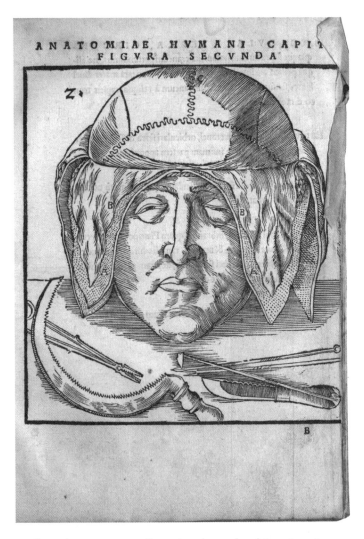

preface, the rector proudly pointed out that his university was conducting public anatomies hitherto neglected in the German lands, and which marked the restoration of the pristine study of anatomy to its honoured place. It served as an advertisement for

19 Dissection of the head with an 'orbicular saw' and other instruments. Dryander, *Anatomy of the Head* (1536). Page height *c.* 20 centimetres/7⅞ in.

the University of Marburg that was recently founded in 1527 by Philip of Hesse (1504–1567).

This book, and an expanded edition in 1537, were among numerous tracts on medical and mathematical topics of medium size (page height *c.* 20 centimetres/7⅞ in.) that Dryander began publishing from 1535 on becoming professor at Marburg, and aimed at the student market or local practitioners. Such a series of publications helped to build a solid local reputation and led him to become a figure of authority whom Philip of Hesse consulted on various matters, including scrutiny of Hans Staden's account of his captivity by the Tupinambá.[42]

Though published in the same year and of a similar size (page height *c.* 21 centimetres/8¼ in.), Niccolò Massa's *Introductory Book on Anatomy* was different from Dryander's book in that it had no illustrations and was bulkier (216 pages).[43] Born in Venice, Massa acquired his degree in surgery from the College of Physicians in 1515. The Venetian College had the power to grant medical qualifications and degrees though it did not offer the requisite courses for such qualifications since such teaching was offered nearby at Padua. Its degrees were cheaper than Padua's, which made it attractive to Italians seeking a medical qualification rather than the accolade of a degree from the more famous Padua or Bologna.[44] Massa most likely studied medicine at Padua before obtaining a degree in arts and medicine from the Venetian College in 1521. It also organized annual anatomies in which Massa sometimes participated.

Massa's *Introductory Book on Anatomy* (1536), printed in roman type, was addressed to 'all students of medicine and philosophy'.[45] It was dedicated to Pope Paul III (1468–1549), to whom Copernicus would address his book seven years later. The occasion for writing the book, according to Massa, was his chance encounter with some distinguished fellow physicians revered by common folk but totally ignorant of anatomy. Not only was anatomy necessary for medical students and his ignorant colleagues so that they could deal with injuries or ailments, Massa also underscored the value of anatomy more generally as a way to 'know thyself' – a reference to the words inscribed in the temple of Apollo at Delphi (according to the second-century author Pausanias). While showing himself conversant with the classical works of medicine and literature, and emphasizing the human body as God's creation, Massa eschewed 'gratuitous insults' against Arabic authors or inveighing against those who had made mistakes. No human was free from error. He loved 'truth more than the authorities of men', and the latter should be corrected by anatomical knowledge acquired through skilful dissection. Massa said that he was the first since Avicenna to demonstrate the fleshy panicle (*panniculus carnosus*) and invoked his learned friends and physicians as witnesses. Though acknowledging that Galen had suggested otherwise, Massa followed Mondino's order of dissection through the lower, middle and upper venters, and chose features that could be examined in a single cadaver. The descriptions were based on his own experience and included discussion of Greek terminology as well as references to authors such as Galen and Avicenna. He offered some striking tips for dissection – hanging a cadaver upside down by one leg helped the dissection of the anal area to locate hemorrhoidal veins, for instance. Using eyeglasses (*oculariis*) under candlelight might help to view the *rete mirabile*, which was 'almost imperceptible'.[46] Massa ended his book by repeating the point that he followed truth rather than the authority of others.

Like Benedetti before him, Massa considered anatomy a topic that should interest the cultural elite of Venice. His dedication did not lead to a papal appointment. In contrast, another physician, Girolamo Fracastoro, who dedicated a book on astronomy (*Homocentrica*, 1538) to the same pope, and who already had strong political connections via the Bishop of Verona, secured a papal appointment in 1545.[47] Anatomy was but one topic that Massa

covered in his publications. He published a collection of his letters
in 1550 (augmented in 1558) written learnedly to fellow physicians, academics and noble patients that spanned a range of topics,
including the 'French disease' (as syphilis was then known),
various forms of fever, specific illnesses for which his opinion
had been sought and various other non-medical matters. The
collection showed Massa as a physician with a wide range of competence (one of which was anatomy) who was just as comfortable
discussing medical treatment as he was commenting on philosophical and literary topics, such as the immortality of the soul
and the uses of rhetoric. It demonstrated Massa as a physician
with comprehensive medical expertise and wider learning, which
helped him garner cultural respectability in Venice.[48] He died in
Venice an affluent man, having invested the income from his
practice wisely in properties, bonds and businesses.

THE BOOKS DISCUSSED ABOVE were not the only ones printed
on anatomy in this period.[49] Books on anatomy were still less
numerous than those on other medical topics and they tended
to be of a modest size (page height *c*. 20–22 centimetres/7⅞–
8½ in.), roughly the same as a page of this book. Vesalius learned
much from these books, even if he did not acknowledge them
explicitly. Anatomical terminology could be updated, with words
derived from Greek replacing those derived from the Arabic,
as Benedetti had done; dissection could correct the words of the
ancients and woodcuts could help physicians as well as artists,
Berengario claimed; Dryander showed how sequential images
were an effective way of presenting stages of dissecting the
head; Galen was not infallible and it was better to strive for
'truth' rather than follow an authority slavishly, Berengario and
Massa wrote; Benedetti, Berengario and Massa believed that
the status of anatomy would be improved with the support of

the non-medical elite who could be cited as witnesses and guarantors of anatomical knowledge. These books incorporated humanist scholarship and had the 'look' of humanist learning, while some also included woodcuts. Alongside other books they published, works on anatomy helped to enhance or consolidate the authors' reputation, but there was no dramatic sea change in their careers solely because of their publication on anatomy. Vesalius's book would be much larger, and with it, he pulled off something that none of the others achieved with their books on anatomy.

THREE

Vesalius and the World of Books

ndreas Vesalius was born in 1514 to Isabel Crabbe and Andries van Wesel, an apothecary who served Emperor Maximilian I, Charles V's grandfather.[1] Andries's profession as an apothecary was not as illustrious as that of his father, Everard, who had been physician to the young Maximilian, or that of his grandfather Johannes, who was professor of medicine at the University of Louvain and physician to Charles the Bold, Duke of Burgundy (Maximilian's father-in-law). Perhaps this was because Andries was Everard's illegitimate son, which at the time carried legal and social limitations. All of Andries's children ended up in the 'family' tradition of medical service: Nicolas became an apothecary, Francis was expected to pursue a career in law but became a 'plague doctor' in Vienna and died there, and Anna married the chief barber to Charles V. Andreas was also destined for a medical career. In 1531, a year after he entered university, his father was legitimized by the emperor and made his 'valet de chambre'. This was an official recognition of Andries's status as a member of the imperial court and as an apothecary.

On the frontispiece of *Fabrica* (illus. 1), Vesalius made the point that he was from Brussels – the location of the imperial court. In the preface, he made clear that his father was in imperial service and that his mother was in a position to acquire an imperial privilege for his book. By the time he was writing *Fabrica*,

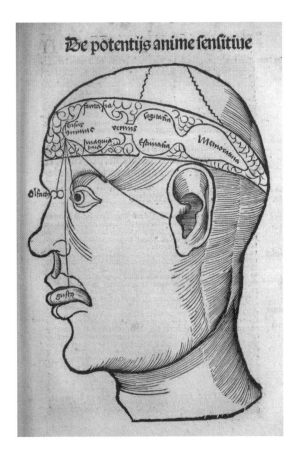

he knew that books were a way to demonstrate learnedness and a means of social advancement. In this chapter, I trace his entry into this world of books.

VESALIUS ENTERS THE WORLD OF PRINTED BOOKS

After being schooled in Brussels, Vesalius matriculated at the University of Louvain in 1530, where he must have been taught a conventional, bookish course in the arts curriculum. Vesalius

20 Figure of the Aristotelian internal senses, from Reisch, *The Pearl of Philosophy* (1503). The young Vesalius and his friends were taught that this image 'showed all parts of the head combined, not just the brain'.

rarely commented on his own education, but one of the books
he mentioned from his time at Louvain was Gregor Reisch's *The
Pearl of Philosophy*, which covered all the subjects taught in an arts
curriculum.[2] Vesalius commented disparagingly on one of its
figures (illus. 20). It illustrated the 'sensitive' soul, one of the three
functions (vegetative, sensitive and intellective) assigned to the
soul (that is, what animated the body) in Aristotelian philosophy. It was posited that within the sensitive soul there were, as
shown in Reisch's figure, 'internal' senses that processed perceptions from the five external senses of sight, hearing, smell, taste
and touch. Located in different parts of the ventricles of the brain,
the 'common sense' gathered sense perceptions, the 'imaginative'
sense combined them, the 'estimative' sense assessed them, and
the 'memorative' sense at the back of the head remembered and
recalled them.[3]

Reisch's woodcut combined diagrammatic and figurative
features. The lines from the ear, eye, nose and tongue converging
at the front ventricle marked the common sense (*sensus communis*).
This indicated that all perceptions from the external senses were
received there, though it is not obvious how this process occurred
anatomically. In contrast, the curled pattern surrounding the
outline of the ventricles suggests the cortical convolutions of
the brain and the jagged lines at the top of the head indicate the
sutures of the skull.

The soul and its workings had long been of interest to theologians. Thomas Aquinas (1224–1274) and John Duns Scotus
(1265/6–1308), for example, had discussed to what extent operations of the internal senses were shared between humans and
animals. It was also a theologian who taught Reisch's textbook at
Louvain, and whom Vesalius criticized for assuming that the
figure showed all that there was to know about the entire head.[4]
While Reisch's figure came to represent for Vesalius the ignorance
and arrogance of theologians, it had also made an impression on

him. As a student, he was told to copy it, and students who were keen to draw copied it carefully into their own notes. This is an intriguing anecdote about the role of drawing in the process of note-taking. We alas do not have Vesalius's drawings from his youth. We do not otherwise know how he might have been trained in drawing, though we know that he drew during his anatomies.

In 1533, at the recommendation of Nicolas Herco Florenas, one-time teacher of Greek, physician to Charles V and godfather to his brother Nicolas,[5] Andreas enrolled in the faculty of medicine at Paris, the most prestigious university for medicine north of the Alps. Paris is where Vesalius saw first-hand the 'successful rebirth of medicine', as he put it.[6] The faculty had already acquired the Aldine edition of Galen in Greek.[7] Jacques Dubois (Sylvius in Latin) was lecturing on Galen to a large crowd of students, using images and actual body parts of animals, while Johann Guenther von Andernach was translating the works of Galen into Latin from the original Greek, and revising other humanist translations of Galen.[8] At Paris, Vesalius discovered that he was good at dissecting, and learned what humanist medical books looked like. His time in Paris overlapped with that of those who would soon become better known, such as the surgeon Ambroise Paré (c. 1510–1590), the Protestant reformer Jean Calvin (1509–1564), the founder of the Society of Jesus Ignatius of Loyola (1491–1556), and the heretic and discoverer of pulmonary circulation Michael Servetus (1511–1553). There is no direct evidence that Vesalius knew these men while in Paris. He would meet Paré later at Henri II's deathbed.

Vesalius began assisting Dubois in his dissection of animals, as well as in the private and public dissections by Guenther.[9] Among those whom he dissected was a beautiful prostitute who had been hanged.[10] He kept in his room 'for weeks on end' body parts obtained from dissections or elsewhere for improving his skills and knowledge. He visited the gallows at Montfaucon, observed sufferers of elephantiasis at the leprosarium of Saint-Lazare, and spent many hours at the Cemetery of the Innocents studying bones with his compatriot Matthaeus Terminus.[11] His familiarity with the city was slipped into *Fabrica*: the intestines had different names for their parts despite being one organ, just like the road between Porte Saint-Jacques and Porte Saint-Martin which had no fewer than six different names.[12]

By the time Vesalius had arrived in Paris, Guenther had published his Latin translation of Galen's *On Anatomical Procedures* (1531), dedicated to Francis I, the king of France. This version swiftly superseded Berengario's edition of Chalcondyles's translation. It was printed by Simon de Colines, who also made his own punches for casting types hailed as 'the first coherent and aesthetically satisfying' set of roman and italic types north of the Alps (illus. 21).[13] Colines' types were certainly appropriate for humanist editions and cemented the wider adoption of roman type in academic publication. Roman majuscules were used for the title of each section and a large decorative initial started each chapter. Just as in the Aldine Galen (illus. 13), the margin was used to number the lines – every five lines in Colines' case – which in turn were used in the index to pinpoint a word on the page.[14]

The book (page height *c.* 35 centimetres/13¾ in.) also had a title page designed by Geoffroy Tory, a type-designer and printer (illus. 22). The title page had been used in the previous year for a translation of Galen's *Method of Healing* by the humanist Thomas Linacre. Its pictorial motifs suggest that it was meant for both editions.[15] In the woodcut, the name of the author and the title of the book are presented in the centre on a tablet, with decreasing size of roman capitals, followed by Guenther's name (in Latin form) in italics, and at the bottom the place, printer and year of publication. The tablet is flanked by Asclepiades, a Greek physician (late second to early first century BCE), and Dioscorides, a Greek author (first century CE) of a book on medicinal materials. Further themes and figures are placed in a three-tiered architectural structure with four Corinthian columns. At the top tier in the centre is a scene from the Old Testament of Job afflicted with boils. On either side of this scene are the twin patron saints of physicians, Cosmas and Damian, the former holding a book and the latter a urine flask. In the middle tier between the columns, the Greek medical authorities are figured: Hippocrates, Galen, Paul of Aegina (active *c.* 630 CE) and Oribasius

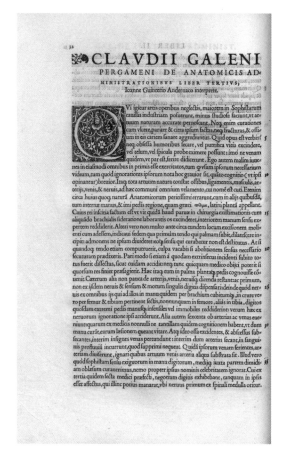

21 Guenther's translation of Galen's *On Anatomical Procedures* (1531), with line numbers marked in the interior margin. Page height *c.* 36 centimetres/14 in.

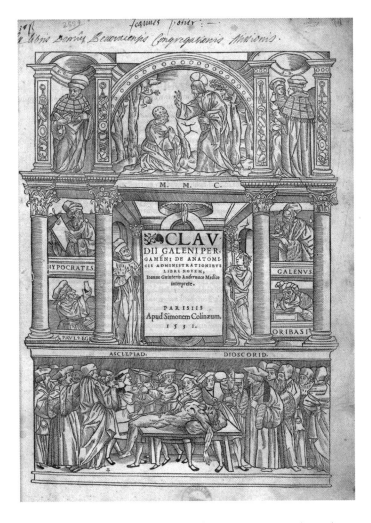

(*c.* 325–400 CE). At the bottom is a dissection scene, with a cadaver
in the centre, surrounded by a crowd of men in academic berets
and robes with trims, gesturing to each other. In the middle is a
youngish man with one hand reaching into the body and the other
pointing upwards, as if to make a point of argument. It is quite

22 Title page of Guenther's translation of Galen's *On Anatomical Procedures*
(1531), with a Lorraine cross (bottom, left of centre), Geoffroy Tory's mark.

possible that this full-page architectural image with a scene of dissection was another inspiration for *Fabrica*'s frontispiece.

Guenther's translation of *On Anatomical Procedures* was also printed in the same year at Basle by Andreas Cratander, a printer known for publishing scholarly books in Greek and in Latin. Several other books published by Colines were published almost simultaneously in Basle. This arrangement helped books reach a wider market, as printers in Basle had better commercial networks across the Holy Roman Empire.

Similarly, Guenther's textbook on Galenic anatomy, *Principles of Anatomy according to the Opinion of Galen, for Medical Candidates*, first printed by Colines in a small format (page height 15 centimetres/ 6 in.) was also printed in Basle, but not by Cratander, who was retiring. The printing was undertaken by a new partnership of Thomas Platter and Balthasar Lasius, who had bought part of Cratander's business.[16] It was a textbook aimed at students, incorporating Galen's *On Anatomical Procedures* and *On the Usefulness of the Parts*, though it was arranged in the Mondinian order of dissection. Latin anatomical names derived from the Greek were used in the main text, with the corresponding traditional names derived from the Arabic placed in the margins. This was a transitional textbook designed to meet the expectations of an academic audience accustomed to Mondino's book and its Arabic-derived terminology and at the same time update it with the latest humanist scholarship.[17] It also marked Vesalius's debut in print, as he was cited by Guenther for discovering that the seminal arteries initially follow a different course from the seminal veins, a point unknown to ancient writers: 'Andreas Vesalius, the son of the apothecary to the Emperor Charles, by Hercules, a young man of great promise, and, in addition to his singular knowledge of medicine, learned in both languages [Greek and Latin], and extremely dexterous in dissecting bodies.'[18] It had not escaped Guenther's notice (perhaps Vesalius made sure of that) that Vesalius's father was in imperial service. These words nicely capture the two important aspects of Vesalius's medical education at Paris: humanist studies and dissection.

When war broke out in 1536 between Charles V and Francis I, Vesalius's family connection to the emperor must have made it prudent for him to leave Paris. He went back to Louvain to complete his medical studies. While there, he made an articulated skeleton by stealing body parts from the gallows with a friend, the mathematician and astronomer Gemma Frisius. In this period, bodies of the executed were often left outside the city walls as a reminder to the public of the consequences of crime. Vesalius noted that the birds had picked off the flesh of the executed cadaver, just as Galen had described the body of a murdered brigand in *On Anatomical Procedures*.[19] Galen had advocated the study of the human body whenever the opportunity arose, and this episode conveyed the point that Vesalius was making as much an effort as Galen had. A fully articulated human skeleton must have been relatively rare at this time, as it impressed the burgomaster of Louvain, Adriaan van Blehen (according to Vesalius) so that he granted more corpses for anatomy. The skeleton itself was left at the home of his childhood friend and physician Gisbertus Carbo.[20] It was a reminder of his presence at Louvain and material proof of his manual dexterity.

Here Vesalius compiled his first book, a small tract (page height *c.* 15 centimetres/6 in.) entitled *The Paraphrase of the Ninth Book of Rhazes, on the Cure of Diseases of Every Part of the Body by the Author Andreas Vesalius, Candidate in Medicine*, which was printed in February 1537 by Rutgerus Rescius, a teacher of Greek who also published Greek texts.[21] At this time, it was neither obligatory nor common for those who were about to obtain a medical doctorate to publish a dissertation, and it suggests a self-awareness on Vesalius's part to distinguish himself from other ambitious medical candidates and get ahead in the world of learned medicine.

From Schedel's list of lectures, we know that Rhazes's book was one of the standard university texts read by professors of practical medicine. It listed diseases by the parts of the body affected, from head to toe, describing symptoms and remedies for each. Vesalius's version was dedicated to the family friend and imperial physician, Florenas.[22] There was another family connection as it was a text on which his grandfather Everard had written a commentary.[23] Vesalius's commentary on a medieval Arabic author might look disappointing in light of his exposure to humanist scholarship in Paris, but he cited Dubois' estimation of Rhazes as 'first among the Arabs' in offering something useful for practical medicine.[24]

The title 'paraphrase' suggested a classical treatment of the text. The Roman rhetorician Quintilian (c. 35–100 CE) recommended 'paraphrase' as a way of learning another's text, not as a slavish summary, but as an active form of intervening in the text by adding what was missing or paring down what was superfluous in the original.[25] It was a format that enabled Vesalius to transform the entire text for the better by removing 'barbarous' medical terms and making corrections using Greek authorities, which Vesalius noted was also the way Parisian physicians approached the text.[26]

Vesalius's paraphrase had the typical humanist feature of correcting a work that had been written later than the ancient Greeks by using knowledge of the Greeks. The main text was printed in a single column in roman type. Medieval Latin terms, many of which were derived from the Arabic, were replaced with Greek words printed in Greek type, with marginal annotations indicating alternative medicines, dosages or treatment suggested by Galen, Paul of Aegina, Aetius, Theophrastus, Pliny the Elder and Celsus, as well as by more recent humanist authors such as Leoniceno. Different types of textual intervention were demarcated with typographical symbols. A clover mark against an Arabic

word (transliterated into Latin) in the main text was a cue for
equivalent words in Greek or Latin under the same mark in the
margin; a set of brackets indicated lengthier comments inserted
in the text; and a dagger indicated variant readings of Rhazes's
text.[27] This was a traditional university text updated with humanist
techniques by a candidate for a medical degree, and dedicated to
a physician at the court of Charles v.

Just like his teacher Guenther, Vesalius had his *Paraphrase* printed
also in Basle, dated later in the same year, 1537.[28] It was printed
by Robert Winter, a publishing partner of Lasius and Platter. In
this edition of *Paraphrase*, the phrase 'medical candidate' was dropped
from the title page, and Vesalius was now simply identified as its
author. The Basle edition is of a similar size to the Louvain version,
printed also in roman and Greek types, and included corrections
to the earlier text. The typographical symbols used to mark
Vesalius's comments were different in the Basle edition, reflecting
the availability of different types. It also had a new 'index of memorable words and things' (illus. 23), another sign of Vesalius's
awareness of humanist sensibilities, since identifying appropriate
classical words for objects was another way in which humanists
hoped to improve knowledge.[29] The woodcut initial decorated
with a kneeling putto holding a staff at the head of the index was
originally designed by Hans Holbein the Younger (1497–1543)
for the printer Cratander, whose business Winter's partnership
had purchased.[30]

In entering the world of printing, *Paraphrase* was the book
on which Vesalius cut his teeth. Proofreading carefully, visually
demarcating the text to clarify different levels of commentary,
compiling an index of 'memorable words and things' that listed
topics he had commented on, and a decorative initial with putto
were all elements that were carried over into his *Fabrica*.

At some point, a decision must have been made, perhaps on
the advice of Florenas, that Vesalius ought to obtain his medical

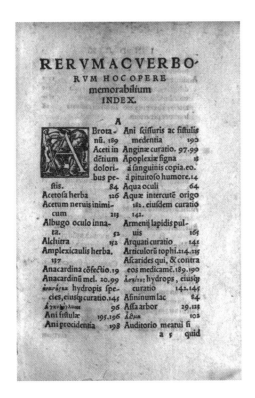

RERVMACVERBO-
RVM HOC OPERE
memorabilium
INDEX.

A

Brota- Ani fciffuris ac fiftulis
nũ. 189   medentia   190
Aceti in Anginæ curatio. 97.99
dētium Apoplexiæ figna   13
dolori-   à fanguinis copia.eo.
bus pe-   à pituitofo humore.14
ftis.   84 Aqua oculi   64
Acetofa herba   126 Aquæ intercutē origo
Acetum neruis inimi-   182. eiufdem curatio
cum   213   142.
Albugo oculo inna-   Armenij lapidis pul-
ta.   52   uis   165
Alchitra   152 Arquati curatio   141
Amplexicaulis herba.   Articulorũ tophi.214.215
137   Afcarides qui, & contra
Anacardina cõfectio.19   eos medicamē.189.190
Anacardinũ mel. 20.99 Ασκίτης hydrops , eiusꝗ
ασκιτικα hydropis fpe-   curatio   142.145
cies,eiusꝗ curatio.145 Afininum lac   84
ἀγκυλόβλωσα   96 Affa arbor   29.125
Ani fiftulæ   195.196 λέμα   102
Ani procidentia   198 Auditorio meatui fi
a 5   quid

degree outside Louvain. It was fairly common, for financial or other reasons, to obtain a degree from an institution different from one's place of study in this period. Felix Platter, the printer Thomas Platter's son, took his degree in Basle after studying at Montpellier despite the fact that Basle's medical faculty was not as renowned as Montpellier's, for example. This was because he was planning a medical career in Basle and the local academic connections mattered more to him.[31] Vesalius's career aspirations went the other way. Rather than embedding himself in a local academic community, he was hoping for a degree with a Europe-wide appeal and distinction – a degree from 'the world's most renowned university', as he called Padua.[32] This may account

23 'Index of memorable things and words in this work', with an initial of a kneeling putto, designed by Hans Holbein the Younger and cut by Jacob Faber. Vesalius, *Paraphrase* (Basle, 1537). Page height *c.* 15 centimetres/6 in.

for the two editions of his *Paraphrase*. Publication of a textbook marked as by a candidate for a medical degree and printed in Louvain might have persuaded academics in Louvain that its author was of a sufficient standard to obtain a degree there. A Basle publication and the erasure of his status as a medical student would have made the book less specifically tied to Louvain. Vesalius was soon headed for Padua.

VESALIUS GOES TO PADUA

The Republic of Venice was actively involved in the administration of the University of Padua from the beginning of the fifteenth century.[33] The Venetian patriciate who formed the hereditary oligarchy of the republic studied at Padua before embarking on their political career, and many developed a personal and active interest in intellectual matters as well as affairs of the university.[34] After the War of the League of the Cambrai (1509–17) in which Padua fought against Venice and lost, the republic increased its control over the university. Three Venetian senators were appointed to oversee all aspects of the university, including appointments. Their efforts in the 1530s indicate an interest in keeping Padua up to date with the latest scholarly developments. The university tried in vain to attract the Greek scholar and professor of medicine at Ferrara, Giovanni Manardi, who was famed for his scholarship on medical terminology and botany. The lectureship on medicinal plants set up in 1533 for Manardi was eventually filled by a Paduan, Francesco Bonafede, who would go on to request the founding of a medical garden in 1543. Existing professors such as Franciscus Frigimelica lectured on the medical botany of Dioscorides, and Giunio Paolo Crasso published a Latin translation of the Byzantine Greek physician Theophilus of Aquasparta's *On the Fabric of the Human Body* (1536), which summarized Galen's *On the Usefulness of the Parts*.[35]

Competition from the Venetian College of Physicians was also intensifying. It had been undercutting Padua with lower fees to the point that between September 1538 and February 1539 no medical degrees (but 26 law degrees) were awarded at Padua. This was followed by the award of six medical degrees between February and June 1539, all with discounted fees.[36] In 1539, Padua persuaded Giovanni Battista da Monte to move from Ferrara to its first ordinary professorship in practical medicine. Though he had hardly published, da Monte had a reputation as a humanist scholar and a teacher of practical medicine. At Padua, he enhanced bedside teaching at the Hospital of St Francis following Galenic principles of classifying and identifying diseases.[37] It is amid this general trend of promoting humanist scholarship in medicine that Vesalius arrived in Padua.

We do not know exactly when Vesalius reached Padua. He had completed his studies at Paris and Louvain, which must have been recognized by Padua as he was permitted to proceed to his examination, and was awarded his doctorate in medicine on 5 December 1537.[38] He was promptly appointed to occupy both posts in surgery and began a public anatomy on 6 December which lasted until 24 December. We should not overestimate this appointment as an endorsement of Vesalius's greatness, since he was still relatively unknown. The salary of the professor of surgery (20 florins per annum) was always acknowledged as low, and thus the statutes allowed for the two professorships in surgery to be held by one person. This was the case in 1529, when Nicolò de Musicis was appointed to both posts, and three years later, in 1532, his salary was increased to 60 florins.[39] When Vesalius was appointed to occupy both professorships in surgery for a total of 40 florins, it was therefore not a particularly exceptional arrangement. Nor was the increase of his salary to 70 florins two years later.[40]

Vesalius was both overqualified and underqualified for the post. The professorship of surgery did not require a medical

doctorate (which Vesalius had just acquired) but did stipulate
a minimum of four years of practice as a surgeon (experience
Vesalius did not have).[41] Yet this appointment did perhaps make
sense in light of the public anatomy conducted the previous year.
In 1536, the two professors of surgery had delegated the task of
dissection (as they were permitted to do) to a Venetian surgeon,
Giovanni Antonio Lonigo, who used Guenther's *Principles of Anatomy*
to guide his dissection.[42] Vesalius had been praised in that book.
He had also shown himself capable of updating a traditional university text with humanist scholarship in his *Paraphrase*. Vesalius's
appointment thus fits the general trend of favouring humanist
scholars at Padua.

The professorship of surgery, however, was at the bottom of
the academic pecking order. In 1537, the salaries paid to the other
professors of medicine were as follows:

First ordinary professor in theoretical medicine	1120 florins
First ordinary professor in practical medicine	500 florins
Second ordinary professor in practical medicine	450 florins
Second ordinary professor in theoretical medicine	400 florins
First extraordinary professor in practical medicine	160 florins
First extraordinary professor in theoretical medicine	90 florins
Second extraordinary professor in practical medicine	85 florins
Second extraordinary professor in theoretical medicine	50 florins
Third extraordinary professor in practical medicine	20 florins
Third extraordinary professor in theoretical medicine	20 florins[43]

The first ordinary professor of theory reigned supreme in rank
and pay. The order of the remaining professors according to their
pay suggests that at this time those teaching practical medicine
were valued a little more than those teaching theoretical medicine
at a comparable rank. Apart from the first ordinary professor of
theory who could not be a Paduan citizen and the first and second

extraordinary professors of theory, the remaining professors (that is, seven out of the ten) were natives of Padua.[44] The most junior of these professors was the third extraordinary professor of practical medicine, who had waited three years after obtaining his doctorate in 1534 to get to the bottom rung of the ladder of academic medicine.[45] Climbing up this ladder took time, even for Paduans. Frigimelica – a Paduan – who presided over Vesalius's doctoral examination as the second ordinary professor in practical medicine had reached that position eleven years after taking his doctorate, and it was at the age of 65 that he was called as papal physician to the deathbed of Pope Julius III (1487–1555).[46]

Vesalius – not a Paduan – was not in the mood for waiting. He started off in 1538 by publishing in Venice a revised version of Guenther's *Principles of Anatomy* for use in his lectures.[47] It was a small booklet (page height 11 centimetres/4⅓ in.) that could easily be carried around and was affordable to students. This was supplemented by the *Anatomical Tables* (1538), a set of six large sheets (page height *c.* 50 centimetres/20 in.) of woodcuts showing the veins, arteries and bones. These were printed in Venice by Bernardino Vitali, who had printed an edition of Berengario's *Isagoge* in 1535. The cost of production was met by the artist Jan Steven van Calcar, whom Vesalius credits explicitly with the creation of the three figures of the skeleton (from the front, side and back) and praised as an outstanding painter of his time.[48] Just as Guenther's *Principles of Anatomy* helped medical students move on to new humanist terminology, the text accompanying the woodcut figures provided the names of parts of the body in Greek, Hebrew or medieval Latin.

The first sheet of *Anatomical Tables* carried a dedicatory text addressed to Narciso Verdú of Naples, chief physician to Charles V, whom Vesalius (or his father) may have met when Verdú came to Brussels accompanying the ambassador of the Kingdom of Naples.[49] The hope, implied by the dedication, that Verdú might mention Vesalius favourably to the emperor was dashed as he was rarely in attendance at court. Instead, as Vesalius later noted in *Fabrica*, his father showed the sheets to the emperor, who viewed it with 'pleasure' and asked 'detailed' questions about it.[50]

The diagrammatic figures of the veins and arteries of Vesalius's *Anatomical Tables* (illus. 24 and 25) presented a Galenic view of the body. The blood vessels roughly formed the shape of the human body, while the liver and the heart were shown in an exaggerated size to indicate their importance as the origin of veins and arteries respectively. According to Galen, the human body was maintained and nourished by the four humours: black bile (produced in the spleen), yellow bile (gall bladder), phlegm (brain) and blood (liver). These four combined to make up the blood that flowed through two different sets of vessels, the veins and the arteries. The veins were understood to originate from the liver (illus. 24) and distribute 'natural spirits' that maintained and nourished the body. The venous blood was believed to seep from the right ventricle of the heart (considered part of the vena cava) into the left ventricle. There, the natural spirit was refined and mixed with the aerial matter delivered from the lungs via the 'veinlike artery' (pulmonary vein) to become the 'vital spirit', which vivified and regulated heat in the body (illus. 25). The vital spirit was carried through the body by the arteries and was refined further in the ventricles of the brain to become the 'animal spirit' required for the working of the internal senses in imagining, reasoning and remembering. Blood was believed to ebb and flow through various parts of the body, where it was consumed as needed. Disease was understood as being caused by stagnation of blood and/or imbalance of humours, which could be rectified by various forms of evacuation, including blood-letting. Despite his anatomical findings, Vesalius's view of the body remained within this humoral framework.

When Vesalius arrived in Padua in 1537, Benedetto Vittori of Faenza was the first ordinary professor of theoretical medicine,

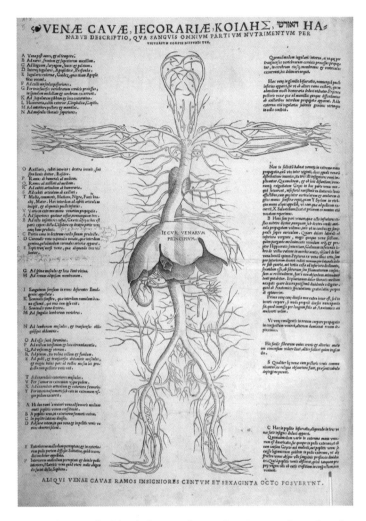

having been called back from Bologna five years earlier after the highest-paid professor of medicine at the time, Matteo Corti, had left Padua to become physician to Pope Clement VII.[51] Vittori had just published *On the Pain of the Side according to the Views of Galen and Hippocrates* (1536), a topic on which his predecessor Corti had

24 'Liver, the source of veins' (inscription on the liver). *Anatomical Tables* (1538). Page height *c.* 50 centimetres/20 in.

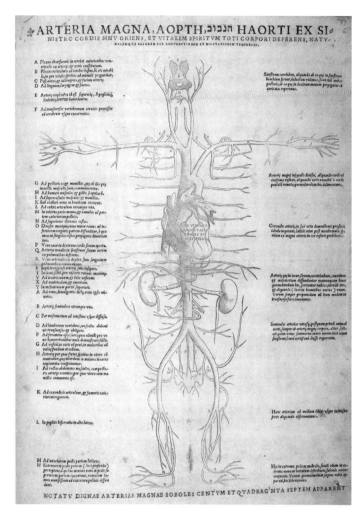

already published twice and was about to publish again in 1538. This concerned the points from which blood should be let in order to remove noxious humours in cases of inflammation of the chest called 'pain of the side'. Originally raised in the 1520s as a therapeutic problem dealing with an outbreak in Evora, by this

25 'Heart, the nurse of the vital faculty and source of arteries' (inscription on the heart). *Anatomical Tables* (1538). Page height *c.* 50 centimetres/20 in.

time 'pain of the side' had become a topic for learned physicians to display their scholarly and humanist credentials about bloodletting. Corti, Vittori and others cited passages by Galen and Hippocrates to endorse a treatment of bloodletting from a point closer to the inflammation rather than from a point farther away, as the Arabic commentators recommended.

It cannot be a coincidence that this was the topic on which Vesalius published next, in 1539, *A Letter Teaching that in Cases of Pain of the Side, the Axillary Vein in the Right Elbow Should Be Cut.*[52] He too discussed relevant passages from Galen, and supported his argument by reference to the anatomical structure of the azygos vein. The tract took the form of a long (66-page) letter addressed to Florenas again, written at the Paduan residence of the sons of Count Gabriel Salamanca of Ortemburg, treasurer to Archduke Ferdinand, the younger brother of Charles V.[53] The imperial connection was made even more explicit as Vesalius claimed that the emperor himself had taken an interest in this topic. Vesalius thus framed his discussion of bloodletting points for a particular affliction into a topic that was far more significant than just a scholarly debate for physicians. This tract was printed not in Venice but in Basle, by Winter again. Vesalius's ambition is clear. By publishing on a topic that the leading professors of medicine at the height of their careers were arguing about, he wanted to show that he could hold his own against those at the top of the academic ladder.

In 1539, da Monte began teaching at Padua with a salary of 500 florins a year. He would go on to occupy the all-important first ordinary professorship in theoretical medicine in 1543 for 700 florins, to be increased to 1,000 florins in 1546.[54] Da Monte was undoubtedly the star professor at Padua at the time. He joined a short-lived group ('the Academy of Burning Ones', *Accademia degli Infiammati*) of philosophers, physicians and others interested in literary and philosophical matters. Vesalius was also acquainted with some of its members, sharing with them a wider interest beyond the confines of medicine.[55] Soon after arriving in Padua, da Monte oversaw the revision of the Latin translations of all the works of Galen for the Venetian publishing firm of Lucantonio Giunta (published 1541–2), who had made a success of publishing Latin translations of Galen.[56] For all the acknowledgement of the importance of mastering ancient Greek, there were many busy learned physicians who were happy to read Galen in Latin rather than plough through the Greek. Da Monte established whether the many tracts attributed to Galen were genuine or spurious, and used Galen's own classification of medicine to group his writings. Vesalius and his English housemate (then still a medical student) John Caius were invited to contribute to the revision of this Latin edition, which was an endorsement of their humanist scholarly abilities.

In *Fabrica*, Vesalius credited da Monte with restoring Galen's works to a 'perfect order' and praised him as a man with near divine 'genius'. However, da Monte had not published much by then, and Vesalius could not resist adding: 'If only some god would ... induce him to allow his other cogitations ... to be published!'[57] For Vesalius, publication was the mark of a learned physician.

VIRTVTI

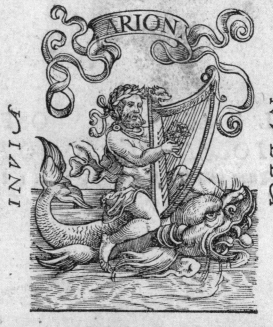

EST VIA

INVIA NVLLA

FOUR

The Making of the Book:
The Printer and the Author

abrica was printed in Basle in the summer of 1543. Its last page carried a printer's mark that Johannes Oporinus (1507–1568) had just began using (illus. 26). It showed the figure of Arion with a lyre – the ancient Greek musician who was robbed and cast off a ship but was rescued by a dolphin attracted to his music. Surrounding the figure is a phrase, 'for virtue there is everywhere a way,' the words spoken by Sybil when Aeneas was about to enter the Underworld, according to the Roman poet Ovid.[1] The woodcut was made by Heinrich Vogtherr the Elder, a versatile craftsman who cut printers' marks as well as decorative initials for various printers.[2] As suggested by his later appointment as oculist to Archduke Ferdinand, Charles v's brother, Vogtherr had some medical background. This may account for his designing and issuing ready-made anatomical paper manikins, consisting of layers of paper cut-outs of the principal organs underneath a flap showing the surface of the body. It illustrated the relative positions of organs inside the body (illus. 27). The paper manikin was a design adopted by Vesalius in both *Fabrica* and *Epitome* (illus. 4), though his were more intricate and accompanied by instructions on how to construct them.[3] Since the woodblocks of *Fabrica* and *Epitome* had been prepared separately in Italy, we can rule out Vogtherr's direct involvement in the production of images for these books. It is also possible that Vesalius came across the idea

26 Johannes Oporinus's mark (7.7 × 6 centimetres/3 × 2½ in.) by Heinrich Vogtherr the Elder.

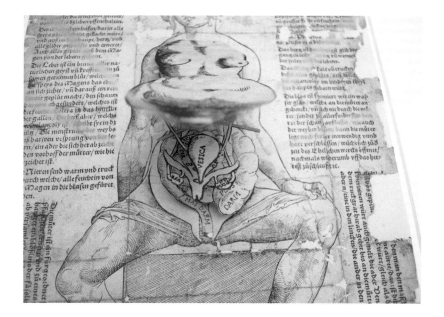

in Italy, as a similar sheet of anatomical flaps was printed in 1539 in Venice.[4] The relationship between the printer and the author was crucial since much co-ordination and care was necessary for bringing about a book like *Fabrica*, as will be discussed in this chapter.

THE PRINTER

The choice of Basle as a place of publication was a little odd for a professor at Padua, whose default printer would have been in nearby Venice because of the local student market and the convenience when overseeing the printing of the book.[5] Vesalius had used Venetian printers for material related to his teaching, namely the *Six Anatomical Tables* and his revised edition of Guenther's textbook. But he had also learned from Guenther the importance of being printed in Basle for better distribution

27 *Anatomy or a Likeness of a Woman's Body, How It Is Shaped Inside* (Strasbourg, 1538), original page 37.5 × 25.6 centimetres/14¾ × 10 in.

through the Holy Roman Empire. His paraphrase of Rhazes's book and the letter on bloodletting had been printed in Basle by Robert Winter. It is probably through Winter that Vesalius met Oporinus, Winter's brother-in-law and business partner.

Oporinus – the Latin transliteration of the Greek equivalent of the German name Herbst – was the son of a Basle painter, Hans Herbst, who also designed illustrative material for printed books.[6] Ambrosius and Hans Holbein the Younger had worked under Herbst, and one of the decorative initials with a putto designed by Hans had been used in the Basle edition of Vesalius's *Paraphrase* (illus. 23).[7] Herbst's son, Johannes, attended university, became proficient in Latin and Greek, and taught at a local school. He also worked for Johannes Froben, an important printer of humanist texts north of the Alps, especially of works by the arch-humanist Desiderius Erasmus (*c.* 1466–1536). Oporinus's work for Froben involved, for example, a transcription of the manuscripts of Irenaeus (second-century Bishop of Lyon), which were then edited by Erasmus.[8] It is probably through Froben that Oporinus met the unorthodox itinerant healer Theophrastus von Hohenheim (later known as Paracelsus), who had saved Froben's gangrenous leg from amputation (though he died soon afterwards).[9] Oporinus served as Paracelsus's assistant and travelled with him for some three years before returning to Basle. When the University of Basle reopened after the turmoil of the Reformation, Oporinus was appointed professor of Latin literature in 1533, and from 1538 he also taught Greek. The university was, however, rocked with controversy when Andreas Bodenstein von Karlstadt, the former and now disaffected colleague of Martin Luther, arrived in Basle and insisted that only those with a doctorate could teach theology, which had not been the case earlier at Basle. Oporinus was actively involved in supporting those against Karlstadt, but they lost their case.[10] He left the university in 1542.

By 1542, Oporinus had become more involved in the printing business. Since 1535, he had been part of a publishing partnership with Lasius, Platter and Winter. To the partnership – as the historian Martin Steinmann aptly summed up – Winter brought the necessary resources, Platter the head for business, Lasius the experience of a compositor, and Oporinus the scholarly nous of obtaining manuscripts and correcting proofs.[11] Oporinus could quite literally correct a Greek manuscript in his sleep – a condition diagnosed as 'waking sleep' by the physician Felix Platter, Thomas's son. Felix related an anecdote that Oporinus, while asleep, had corrected an entire page of a Greek manuscript with his father when they had to pass the night in an inhospitable inn outside the city gates, yet was later unable to recall having done so when he woke up.[12] The partnership's early publications, such as Jean Calvin's *Institutes of the Christian Religion* (1536) and Guenther's *Principles of Anatomy* (1536), listed only the names of Platter and Lasius as the printers. Winter's name appeared for the first time with Vesalius's *Paraphrase* (1537). As corrector of texts, Oporinus was the least visible of the partnership until he acquired his own press.

In the meantime, Oporinus had decided to set up his own press, but he ran into problems almost immediately when he began printing a Latin translation of the Quran, edited by his friend Theodor Bibliander. Bibliander believed that publication of the Quran was essential for converting Muslims to Christianity, and Oporinus sent him an Arabic manuscript from the university library.[13] In the summer of 1542, the Basle authorities halted its printing, and Oporinus was imprisoned. Eventually, Luther's support for the project swayed the city council to permit publication on condition that the place of printing was not marked as Basle. Amid the controversy, Oporinus grumbled about a rumour that 'there was no other place where printing the [Quran] was allowed, and therefore it was pushed on me, a stupid man and a trouble lover.'[14]

Oporinus was far from stupid – in fact, he was considered by his contemporaries as the most learned man in Basle after Erasmus.[15] 'Trouble lover' could be an oblique reference to the fact that he had associated with the controversial Paracelsus. Or, more likely, it was a comment on his part in the dispute at the university. Oporinus was soon released from prison, and the Quran was printed. The motto, 'for virtue there is everywhere a way' (illus. 26), must have rung a personal note of vindication for him. Oporinus was thus a university-educated scholar of Greek and Latin literature who was experienced in printing scholarly works in these languages that demanded careful attention. And, perhaps importantly for Vesalius, he was not averse to taking risks – printing, for instance, a large, scholarly tome with many illustrations.

VESALIUS'S LETTER TO OPORINUS

When Vesalius was writing his letter to Oporinus dated 24 August 1542, he did not know that Oporinus was in prison over the first European printing of the Quran. He addressed his letter to Oporinus as professor of Greek at the University of Basle. Vesalius certainly knew that Oporinus was about to strike out on his own in the printing business 'to the great benefit of scholars'.[16] Some kind of agreement about publishing *Fabrica* and *Epitome* must have been reached prior to this letter.

We do not know when exactly Vesalius began work on *Fabrica* – the earliest is possibly sometime after publication of his *Six Anatomical Tables*, and at the latest after his visit to Bologna in 1540. He not only wrote the text, but also oversaw the preparation of the drawings and the woodcuts. The two known surviving drawings, attributed to Jan Steven van Calcar, were done in red chalk on paper (illus. 28).[17] Though tonally less strong than black chalk, red chalk was less friable and suited to detailed work on a smaller scale on paper, and came to be used more widely in the sixteenth century.[18] The drawings underwent revision under Vesalius's direction to ensure an efficient distribution of anatomical details with limited repetition. Vesalius proudly remarked that the images gave him 'extreme pleasure to look at' and that they were much better than the ones consisting of simple outlines in common schoolbooks – perhaps he had in mind the figure in Reisch's book (illus. 20).[19] The pictorial quality of *Fabrica*'s figures will be discussed in more detail in the next chapter.

The finalized drawings were then traced onto woodblocks which were rediscovered in 1932 before they were destroyed in the bombing of Munich in the Second World War.[20] These blocks were made of pear wood sawn parallel to the grain, as was common at the time. They were possibly treated with hot linseed oil to enable finer cutting. Vesalius oversaw and must have paid for the production of the woodcuts. The occasional mismatch of references to the left or the right between the text and the image suggests that he was sometimes looking at the original drawing rather than the printed image when writing the text.[21]

By the summer of 1542, both the text and the woodcuts were ready. Vesalius began his letter by telling Oporinus that he had packed the woodblocks carefully with the help of an unnamed woodcutter as well as Nicolaas de Stoop (d. 1568).[22] Stoop, from Aalst (northwest of Brussels), worked as corrector for the Venetian printing firm of Daniel Bomberg, who was originally from Antwerp. This hints at an expatriate network of those from the Low Countries (which probably included Jan Steven van Calcar) in Venice which Vesalius could draw on. The woodblocks were sent to Basle by Milanese merchants. They arrived virtually intact. At one point before the printing, one of the blocks developed a pronounced crack in the bottom left corner (illus. 42), which was probably stabilized with some brackets. All surviving copies of *Fabrica* carry this figure with a crack. Vesalius himself arrived in Basle by January 1543, by which time the printing of the

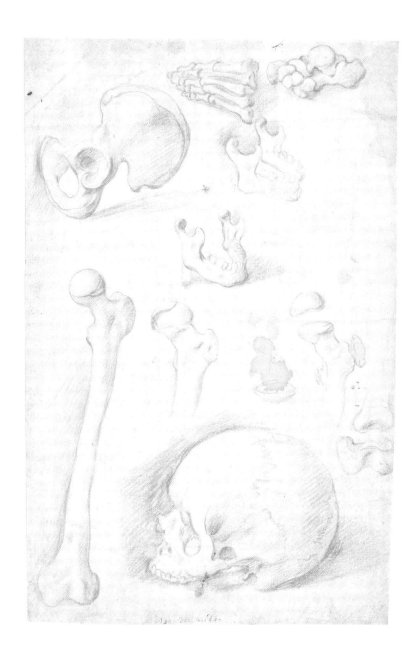

28 Study of bones attributed to Jan Steven van Calcar, red chalk, incised, on cream laid paper, 29.3 × 19.6 centimetres/11½ × 7⅜ in.

book had begun. The printing of *Fabrica* and *Epitome* was completed around July.[23]

Vesalius's letter was a detailed instruction to the printer which also served as an explanation to the readers about the typographical conventions used in the book. Different types were used for the main text (roman) that described anatomical functions and for the morphological descriptions (italics) keyed to the characters in the figures.[24] The characters placed in the figures were chosen from those that were 'in standard use in printing houses': namely, Latin and Greek letters as well as other marks such as ampersands and asterisks (illus. 29). Vesalius had also added a point (or a full stop) after a letter in the description when it was part of a larger structure, thus introducing a distinction of whether a letter denoted an entire structure or not.

Because Vesalius wanted his main description to run without interruption, he made use of the page margins. The outer margin was used (as was common at the time) to indicate the subject covered in the text. The inner margin was for connecting the text with the images. Vesalius asked Oporinus to use 'super-linear' letters next to a word in the text that served as markers in the inner margin for listing the location of relevant images. These cross-references to images in the inner margin were extensive. For example, Book Two alone of *Fabrica* included more than

Γ,Δ *Musculus secundo loco inter scapulam mouentes recensendus. Atqz huius principium ab occi-*
E,F. *pitij osse pronatum, E ac F insignitur. E uerò usqz ad G musculi principium ab occipite, ad*
G. *octauæ usqz thoracis uertebræ spinam, à mediarum uertebrarum apicibus quodammodo enatü.*
H,I. *H, I insertio, quam musculus in scapulæ spinam, & summum humerum, latiusculamqz clauicu-*
＊. *læ sedem molitur. ＊ hac sede præsens musculus, quasi membraneum semicirculum obtinet, seu car*
K. *nosæ ipsius fibræ, in semicirculi cessant circunferentiam. K hac parte ceruix collum ue, thoracis*
elatißimæ parti committitur. Lineæ autem laterá ue musculum circunscribentia in hunc modum
colliguntur. Ab E ad F prima protenditur, ad occiput transuersim ducta. Quòd autem hu
ius extremum F notatum, non tantùm ab auris radice distare hic uideatur, quantùm F remoue
tur ab E pictura, in causa est oculum fugiens, quod & sinistrum brachium in anteriora porre-
ctum liquidò commonstrat, quod forte ὀπﬁκὸς ignarus, plus æquo breuius esse arbitrabitur. Por
rò secunda linea præsentis musculi ab E per K ad G metitur. Tertia autem ab F ad H.
Quarta ab H ad G. Atqz his lineis musculus terminatur. Insertionis autem linea ab I ad
K pertinens, nulla prorsus separationis nota existit.

29 Description in italics of the 'second [trapezius] muscle moving the scapula'), denoted by Greek (ΓΔ), Latin (EFGHIK) and typographic (＊) fonts and full stops, corresponding to keys in the illustration (see illus. 40).

2,000 superscripts (some referring to six to eight illustrations at a time).[25] No wonder Vesalius acknowledged the typesetting in the internal margins as a task that required 'a lot of tedious drudgery'![26] But it wasn't just the typesetters who had to face drudgery. A reader would also have had the cumbersome task of turning the pages back and forth in order to consult all the images listed in the margin. In reading the four-and-a-quarter-page chapter in Book Three (on the blood vessels of the brain), a reader would have been prompted to look up more than a hundred details in various images.[27]

Illustrations too needed to be printed with 'particular care'.[28] Vesalius had sent the proofs with the woodblocks to Oporinus, noting that a clean printing of figures depended on the printer's diligence as well as 'the smoothness and density of the paper'. As a printer, Oporinus did not have a track record in producing lavishly illustrated books, but Vesalius expected him to know what was involved in using woodcuts. This is another sign that Vesalius understood enough of the printing process to know what could make a difference in how the details appeared on the page. He expected no character, 'however hidden in the shading, will escape the notice of the reader', though some of the letters were in fact difficult to locate, as Vesalius himself occasionally conceded.[29]

Vesalius's letter to Oporinus demonstrates the level of attention he devoted to how his book should look. Intriguingly, one visual element that Vesalius did not mention in his letter was the decorative initials.[30] Ornamental initials with naked putti were fairly common in Italy as well as in Basle (illus. 23). In *Fabrica*, large initials with putti equivalent in height to 14 lines of text (of roman type) marked the start of each major section called a 'book'. The large, white-bodied initial Q (illus. 30), used at the beginning of Books One and Five, shows a vivisection of a pig discussed at the end of *Fabrica*.[31] In the lower corners one putto handles a razor similar to the one held by the figure on the ground in front of the dissection table in the frontispiece (illus. 1). Another tests the sharpness of the tip of the tail of Q, suggesting playfully that the letter itself is a physical object with a sharp point. The smaller initials (for example, illus. 51, 65) that were half the height of the larger ones (or the height of seven lines of text in roman type) marked the start of each subsection called a 'chapter'. On one occasion, the decorative initials were used as small illustrations without forming a word. The capital letters E and F (illus. 31) were introduced to show the 'glossocomion' mentioned by Galen which was a wooden encasing with a windlass designed to rectify a dislocated bone.[32] Vesalius here used initials as illustrations rather than letters.

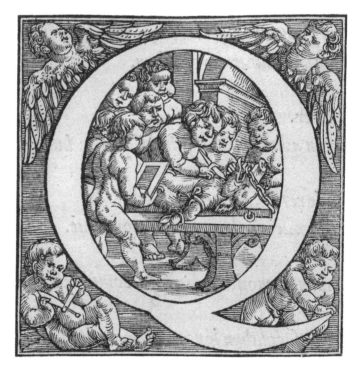

30 Initial Q with a sharp tail. Its height is equivalent to fourteen lines of roman type. 7.5 centimetres/3 in. square.

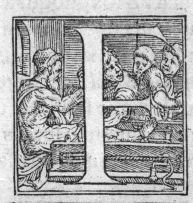

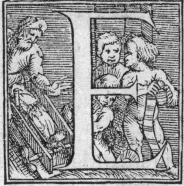

QVONIAM
Galenus in horum neruo,
rum defcriptione, quemad,
modum & nonnunquam a,
libi, mentionem facit inftru
menti gloßicomi, nos lecto
ri non incommodaturos du
ximus, fi hunc charactes
rem F, in quo id inftru,
mentũ obiter exprimitur,
hîc interijceremus: unà cũ
E, quo inftrumentum deli,
neatur brachij, fed potißi,
mum femoris luxationibus
reftituendis idoneum. Li,
cet hæc alio libro ac argu,
mento tractanda pu
temus.

A material product whose every aspect was invested with such care and attention, not to mention cost, was also worth protecting. Vesalius promised Oporinus that he would bring a copy of a decree from the Venetian Senate forbidding unauthorized copying of the illustrations. Printers and authors often paid for legal 'privileges' that protected their product by specifying penalties against unauthorized reprinting and sales. However, since they were valid only in the jurisdiction of the authority issuing them, some, like Vesalius, obtained several. His mother was going to send Oporinus a privilege from the emperor while Vesalius

31 'We thought it no disservice to the reader to insert here the letter F
... together with E in which is shown the instrument suitable to reduce dislocation of the arms and especially the thigh.'

was in the process of acquiring one from the king of France through the mediation of Guillaume Pellicier, Bishop of Montpellier and French ambassador to Venice. Though the existence of these privileges was recorded at the bottom of the title page (illus. 1), Vesalius was sanguine about the efficacy of such a legal instrument as a deterrent against unauthorized copying or plagiarism, as it relied on the wronged party taking the alleged malefactor to court, which could be lengthy and costly.

Vesalius had personal experience of the limited effect of a privilege as a deterrent. His *Anatomical Tables* with a Venetian privilege had been plagiarized poorly several times. One such plagiarizer, Walther Hermann Ryff (*c*. 1500–1548), was well known for compiling books copied from other printed works.[33] He produced a slender anatomical tract (40 pages, *c*. 30 centimetres/11⁴⁄₅ in.) made up of images copied from those in Vesalius's *Anatomical Tables* and elsewhere. In Ryff's work, Vesalius's figure of veins (illus. 24) was superimposed on a seated human body (illus. 32) so that the entire course of veins looked as if they were spread out on the surface of the body, which Vesalius criticized as misleading and absurd. This was a point that needed to be corrected, especially since Vesalius had charged Galen with having seen only the subcutaneous veins in humans. Vesalius certainly did not want to be seen as making the same mistake as Galen.

This is why the figure of veins (illus. 33) in *Fabrica* looks so very different from the ones in *Anatomical Tables* or those in Ryff's tract. The figure in *Fabrica* shows the veins more fully running *throughout* the entire depth and length of the body. In fact, without the outline of the contour of the body, it is the veins alone that form the shape and depth of the human body. The absence of the outline was important to Vesalius:

on no account should they draw an outline around the figure to make it look like another picture of a person;

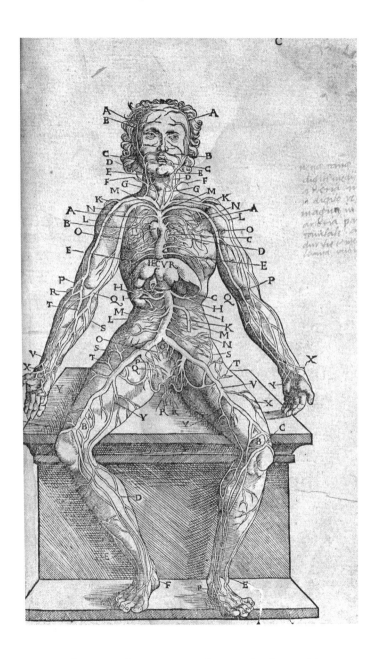

32 Figure of veins in Walter Hermann Ryff, *Anatomy* (1541), copied from *Fabrica* (compare illus. 24).

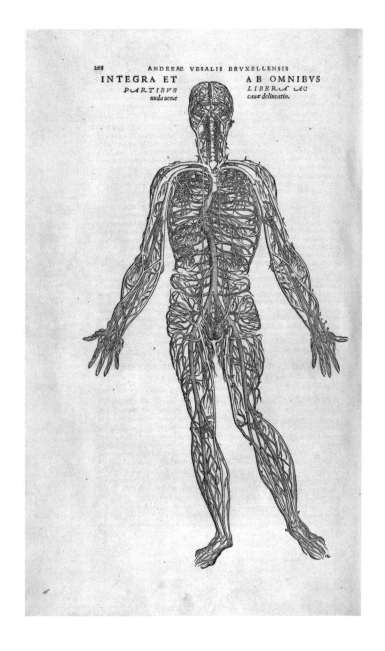

INTEGRA ET   AB OMNIBVS
PARTIBVS   *LIBERA AC*
nuda uenæ   *cauæ delineatio.*

33 '. . . on no account should they draw an outline around the figure
to make it look like another picture of a person.'

some plagiarists actually did this in an edition of my
Anatomical Tables printed in Strasbourg ... Quite apart from
the fact that such an outline spoils the whole effect for a
variety of reasons, it must be rejected because it might
suggest that all the veins portrayed in this figure disperse
into only one surface and belong only to the anterior
portion.[34]

Vesalius's letter to Oporinus underscores the extent of
Vesalius's involvement in the design of the book – its types,
layout, referencing system and figures. Such an involvement
by the author was unusual for the period. This was possible
because of his familiarity with the process of printing through
his earlier publications, and thanks to a printer willing to take
on the challenge.

WORK AT BASLE

Vesalius knew well that instructions to the printer in a letter were
not sufficient to guarantee the desired outcome. He travelled to
Basle to oversee the production since he knew the level of attention
needed during the production process in order to avoid mistakes.
Even with the best proofreaders and correctors, printed books
contained errors, however. These were commonly listed at the
end of the book in 'errata', to be corrected by the readers. Vesalius
was punctilious in his attention to detail, though some evidently
slipped through his net.[35] Textual errors could readily be corrected
by hand by the readers, but mistakes in images were more difficult.
A small woodcut could be added to correct a small section, or a
minor detail could be corrected with a pen by the reader, as Vesalius
suggested, though few readers appear to have obliged.[36]
    Another task that could only be done once the pages had
been printed was compiling the 'index of memorable words and

34 'The reader who has carefully read the work will be able to lengthen the list; we have chosen, because of the authority of Galen, to set down here only a few of the many such passages.'

things', a phrase Vesalius first used in the Basle edition of his *Paraphrase*.[37] The locations of words were given by page and line number in the index, though some of the pages were misnumbered during the printing process. Authoritative texts printed in large formats often included line numbers in their margins (illus. 13 and 21), as did Oporinus's Quran. Although the margins of *Fabrica* were already crowded, it was nevertheless felt appropriate and useful to include line numbers for the purposes of reference, even if it meant that the readers had to count the lines on the page themselves.[38] Of the 34 pages of the index printed in small roman type, three were occupied by more than two hundred entries on Galen. Vesalius remarked that he had chosen 'only a few' as he was sure that his readers could come up with even more examples (illus. 34).[39] In contrast, there were 28 entries on Aristotle, 8 on Hippocrates, 6 on Celsus and 3 each on Plato and Pliny the Elder. Galen was the authority who mattered most to Vesalius. The index also listed in full capital letters Vesalius's friends and supporters whom he mentioned in the text. Vesalius himself appears twice under 'A' (for Andreas), referring to the first skeleton he had articulated at Louvain, and his admonition against the plagiarized copies of his *Anatomical Tables*.[40]

When all was said and done, *Fabrica* was almost seven hundred pages long using paper (height *c.* 43 centimetres/ 17 in.) equivalent to that of a respectable academic tome. The size of the book dignified its content.[41] Even larger were the pages of *Epitome* (page height *c.* 57 centimetres/22½ in., illus. 3). Like Berengario, Vesalius intended his *Fabrica* to have a shorter pictorial version. Though larger in size than *Fabrica*, *Epitome* condensed into eleven pages six short chapters that described the whole body. The text in roman type was printed in double columns, not because Vesalius wanted to emulate the traditional academic look of the page, but because it made it easier to follow the text on an oversized page. Superlinear letters were used again in the main text, but

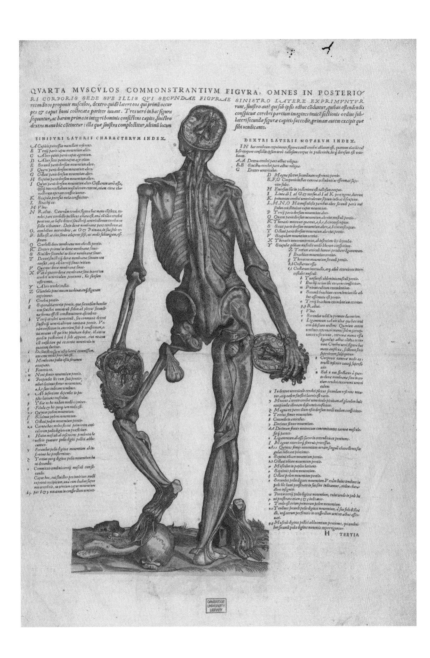

35 Figure four of *Epitome* (1543), epitomizing seven figures from *Fabrica* (1543).

this time to refer to both the inner and outer margins which listed the Greek names of the anatomical parts discussed in the text. *Epitome* used the title page, initials and one of the skeleton figures from *Fabrica*, in addition to its own, larger figures that merged images from *Fabrica*. For example, figure four of *Fpitome* (illus. 35) is an amalgam of table twelve of *Fabrica* (from the knee to the neck on the right side in the figure), table thirteen (from the knee to the neck on the left side), table fourteen (from the knee down, the occipital skull with the vertebrae on the ground and the addiitional foot), and of woodcuts of the brain in three consecutive stages of dissection (the head and the skulls held in each hand).[42] 'Epitome', after all, meant, and still does mean, an abridgement, and that is certainly what the figures did – abridge the images in *Fabrica* to show as many anatomical structures as possible. It also included layered paper manikins for the male and female bodies (illus. 4, 56–9).

Familiarity with printers' work, a scholarly printer willing to take some risk, and proofreading during the printing process were essential elements for staying in control of the end product. Vesalius's earlier experience with publications meant that he could exploit effectively the potentials of the printed page such as typefaces and layout. From the types, full stops and internal and external margins of the page to the woodcuts and the index that carried on his polemic, Vesalius had a clear idea of what his books should look like. Oporinus obliged. Copies of *Fabrica* and *Epitome* materialized from his press in the summer of 1543.

Fabrica and *Epitome* remained the only books with lavish illustrations that Oporinus ever printed. After 1543, his publications focused on the classics and the works of humanists. He also printed and supported heterodox writers such as Sebastian Castellio (who fell out with Calvin and had to leave Geneva) and Guillaume Postel (who was imprisoned in Rome by the Inquisition), and took on the mammoth ecclesiastical history produced from a

Lutheran point of view, the *Magdeburg Centuries* (more than 7,000 pages in multiple volumes, page height *c.* 33 centimetres/13 in.).[43] In contrast to the advantages Vesalius reaped from his books, neither *Fabrica* nor *Epitome* advanced dramatically Oporinus's publishing career.

FIVE

The Human Figure: Art and Anatomy

aldasar Heseler, a student from Silesia completing his studies at Bologna, took notes of the anatomies conducted in 1540 by the visiting professor from Padua, Andreas Vesalius. During his dissection, Vesalius digressed to express his sentiment – shared by many at the time – that the ancients had represented more beautifully the surface muscles of the human body than contemporary artists were able to.

> [Vesalius] only said that the large muscles of the back, the upper arm, the shoulder, etc., which our native artists of today do not paint so beautifully, can be best seen in the ancient monuments and antiquities of the ancient artists. Last year [1539] I saw our artists in Bologna thanks to the grace of the governor taking a plaster cast of a hanged man in the Hospitale alla morte and sketching the superficial muscles, because the doctors at the time did not dissect, for the Rector, an Italian, was ill-disposed and mean.[1]

Vesalius's mention of artists reminded Heseler of an earlier missed opportunity for a public anatomy because of the rector's disinterest, which in turn provided an opportunity for local painters to draw and take casts of the body at the hospital run by the confraternity of St Mary of Death (Santa Maria della Morte) that comforted prisoners and the condemned. Heseler's passing

remark is a reminder of the close proximity in which artists and
anatomists worked, and their shared interest in the human figure,
albeit for different reasons, and with different results. To what
extent did artists depend on knowledge of anatomy to create
a human figure? And to what extent were the images in *Fabrica*
indebted to the artistic culture of the time?

ARTISTS AND HUMAN ANATOMY

It may seem over-fastidious to point out that the Latin word
translated as 'artist' in Heseler's diary above was *pictor*, a painter.
Our modern view of an artist as an embodiment of creative
imagination and talent is indebted to efforts begun in this period
to set the painter apart from other craftsmen.[2] For Leon Battista
Alberti (1404–1472), papal secretary, architect, poet and student
of ancient monuments, statues and inscriptions, this entailed
elevating the craft of painting to a form of knowledge – a liberal
art – valued by the cultural elite. He recast the painter as engaging
his mind – *ingenium* was the Latin word Alberti used – in order
to paint well.[3] In a short tract, *On Painting*, Alberti wrote that knowledge of geometry was fundamental to conveying depth and drawing contours of objects from a fixed point of view; understanding
of how light cast shadows was essential for modelling surfaces;
and familiarity with classical poetry and literature was needed
for compositional elements such as 'grace', 'decorum', 'copious-
ness' and 'symmetry'. To avoid over-relying on the mind, however,
Alberti suggested learning general rules from nature – such as
the relative proportion of parts of the body, the different state of
limbs in dead and live bodies, or the fact that weight placed on one
side of the body was always counterbalanced on the other side
by a leg or an arm.[4] Some knowledge of the underlying structure
of the human body was indeed useful, 'just as when drawing
draperies, one starts with the body underneath, so draw bones

first, then muscles, and then clothes.' He did not, however, advocate
that painters dissect a human body.[5]

Citing the classical precedent of the painter Demetrius who
did not win the highest praise in his time because he was fonder
of expressing likenesses of things than their beauty, Alberti urged
painters to strive for the higher purpose of beauty.[6] Though beauty
was something rarely instantiated in one person, a painter could
learn from nature by selecting the best parts of beautiful individuals. This in itself was a classical idea: the famed painter of antiquity
Zeuxis created a portrait of Helen of Troy by combining the most
beautiful features of five women. Replete with terms of classical
rhetoric and references to classical episodes, Alberti's tract was
thus a self-consciously humanist approach to elevating the art
of painting. While he underscored knowledge of bones and
muscles as valuable for the painter, he did not insist on first-hand
dissection in the way that he insisted painters should know the
principles of geometry. In fact, there is little evidence that Alberti
himself actively took part in dissecting the human body.

Alberti's ideas were familiar to the painter, sculptor and gold-
smith Antonio del Pollaiuolo, known for depictions of muscular
male figures.[7] Yet, his figures were not always anatomically correct,
even though he appears to have encountered some flayed limbs.
Pollaiuolo worked out poses using sculptural models as well as
drawings to help him achieve compositions that looked convincing to a cultural elite who were not known for their precise grasp
of human anatomy. This may be the reason why participation in
dissection was not the most common or commonly available route
for painters or sculptors to study the human body in the fifteenth
century. Familiarity with surface muscles was usually adequate for
representing a plausible human figure. This could be achieved by
sketching family members, apprentices or others going about their
business as well as by studying casts of human limbs. The painter
and sculptor Andrea del Verrochio had casts of human limbs in

his workshop, as did some other Italian painters from the second half of the fifteenth century.[8]

Leonardo da Vinci apprenticed with Verrochio and may have known Alberti.[9] Like Alberti, Leonardo wrote a tract on painting, and he extolled the need for the painter to learn from nature also. Leonardo was fascinated, as was Alberti, with the relative proportions of parts of the body of an ideal human figure, drawing on ideas of the Roman architect Vitruvius (first century BCE). While Leonardo too believed that a painter should be knowledgeable, his interest in the human body went well beyond what was necessary for a persuasive representation of the human figure. He wanted to understand movements and forces in nature and machines. He also dissected humans as well as animals.

At the hospital of Santa Maria Nuova in Florence, Leonardo saw an old man die peacefully sitting up in his bed. Leonardo then dissected his body.[10] This is one of the few cases where we know some details of Leonardo's dissection. It was in fact not unusual for painters to visit hospitals. In the 1490s, the hospital of Ca' Granda in Milan arranged for drawings to be made of private dissections done there by local physicians.[11] Though few painters are recorded as having carried out dissections themselves, hospitals continued to be a place where they could study the human body, as Heseler's remark confirms.

Leonardo's surviving drawings of human anatomy come in a variety of modes: from a detailed study of the papillary muscles in the ventricles of the heart and a drawing of the old man's liver that can be retrospectively diagnosed as suffering from cirrhosis, to a large sketch of a pregnant female amalgamating animal and human dissections with descriptions from books.[12] Leonardo's solution to representing a three-dimensional body and its depth on a two-dimensional page was either to show an object from a number of angles or to reduce muscles to thinner cords so that structures underneath them could be shown in one view

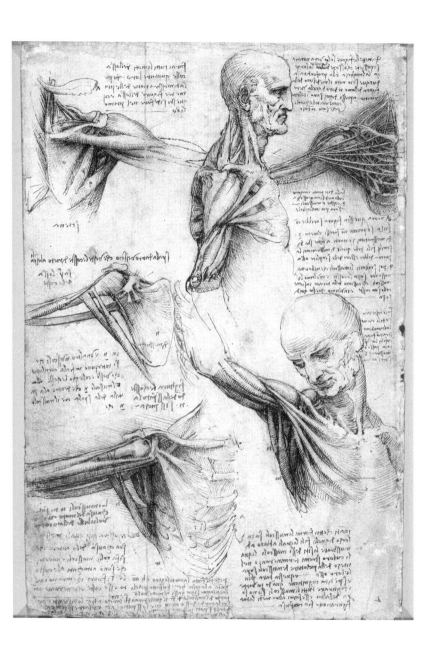

36 Study of muscles of the shoulder by Leonardo da Vinci, c. 1510–11.
Pen and ink with washover black chalk on paper, 29.2 × 19.8 centimetres/
11½ × 7⅘ in.

(illus. 36). We must be careful not to think of these drawings as a documentary record of what Leonardo actually saw or dissected. Leonardo drew to think, imagine, experiment and extrapolate visually about the workings of nature.[13]

Though he did intend to publish a book on human anatomy, this did not come to fruition, possibly because of the shortage of craftsmen capable of creating woodcuts or engravings of the complexity and number he envisaged and the associated expense these would have incurred. Leonardo's anatomical studies remained in private hands and were not generally known in Vesalius's time. A rare verdict came from a contemporary physician Girolamo Cardano, who had seen some of Leonardo's drawings. He deemed them more beautiful than anatomically accurate, noting that Leonardo was more a painter (*pictor*) than a physician (*medicus*).[14]

As Heseler reported, his contemporaries, including Vesalius, thought that classical statues represented the human body better than contemporary painters could achieve. Many of the ancient sculptures unearthed in the Renaissance were of muscular, heroic figures. Artists flocked to Rome to draw them (illus. 2), and casts were made to enable study without having to do so on site. Studies of classical sculptures were not always an inch-perfect imitation of the original sculptures, however: missing limbs could be added and poses could be modified. These were among various other sources of inspiration for compositions involving the human figure in the Renaissance.[15]

A reverence for classical sculpture did not necessarily clash with an empirical study of the human body. This point is illustrated by Michelangelo's study of the Belvedere Torso (illus. 37), which in turn served as a model for his sculpture *Victory*, now at the Palazzo Vecchio, Florence. According to the art historian James Elkins, it is impossible to tell apart in this drawing the parts that were drawn after a dissected cadaver, an antique model or a live body: 'without knowledge of the ribs, Michelangelo could not have depicted their

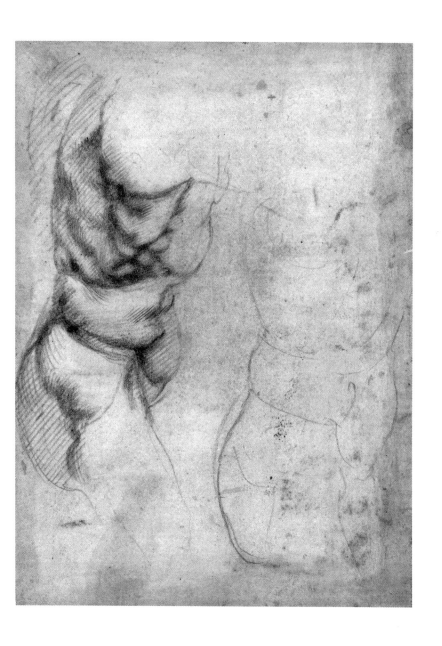

37 Two studies of a male torso in profile by Michelangelo, 1519–23.
Black chalk on paper, 22.5 × 16.5 centimetres/8⅞ × 6½ in.

distortions so fluently or coherently and without having known the Belvedere Torso he would not have arrived at many of the forms of the drawing.'[16] This is another example of why an artistic drawing is not a good source for gauging the extent or accuracy of an artist's anatomical knowledge. For just as Alberti extolled the importance for the learned painter to go beyond mere life-likeness, drawings were an expression of a particular artist's conception (called *disegno* in the period) of what the human figure should look like, based on their training as well as their own inventiveness. When painters did study the human body, it was ultimately subservient to artistic expression. Their primary goal was not the elucidation of the inner workings of the human body.

FABRICA AND ARTISTS

We do not know if Vesalius had read Alberti's tract on painting, which was first published in Basle in Latin in 1540 based on a manuscript that was possibly known to Dürer.[17] Yet, just like Berengario, Vesalius believed that he should edify painters and sculptors for whom he had specifically included the first and second tables of 'thick-set' figures (illus. 38 and 39).[18] The extended and raised arms in these figures illustrated an 'axiom' they should follow: a muscle becomes shorter, more prominent and bunched up around the middle of its belly when pulling a bone towards it, and is lengthened and flattened when it releases the bone. There were also some common pitfalls for even the 'experienced painters and sculptors' who might think that the 'muscle raising the arm' (*musculus deltoideus*, M in illus. 39) was more than one muscle because of its depressions, or assume that the insertion of the 'posterior muscle of those that flex the forearm' (*musculus brachialis*, N in illus. 39) is higher along the outside of the forearm than it should be.[19] Vesalius thus hoped that artists would benefit from knowing some human anatomy.

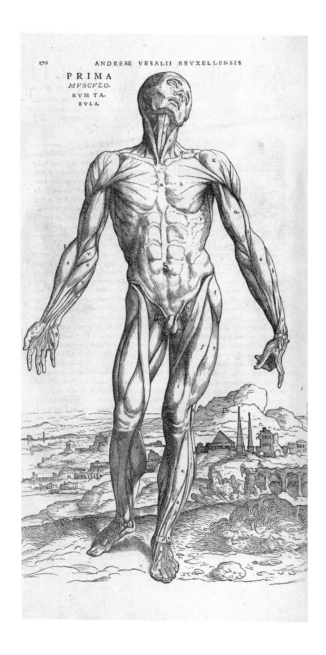

PRIMA
MVSCVLO-
RVM TA-
BVLA.

38 'The first and second [tables] show nothing which we have not every day seen erudite painters and sculptors portray in muscular, and, as I might say, thick-set figures.'

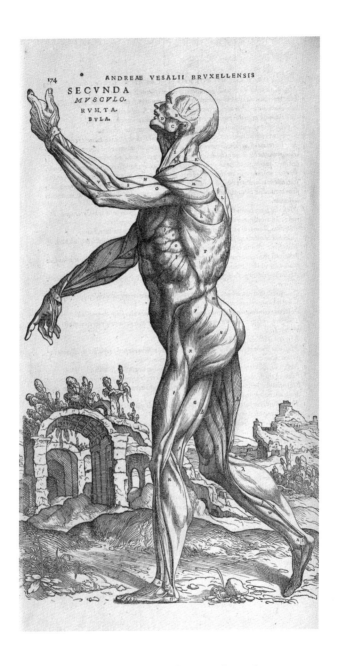

39 'This muscle [M] is more likely than any other to deceive
experienced painters and sculptors, whom I would have pay close
attention not only to this area, but the whole outside of the arm.'

Even these woodcuts that were designed to teach artists had to be made by artists. In a period when there were no professional scientific illustrators, Vesalius relied on the skills of existing painters and woodcutters. We do not know for certain who they were. Less than a handful of original drawings for *Fabrica* have survived, none of which bears a signature (illus. 28). They have been attributed to Jan Steven van Calcar partly because of his involvement in the earlier *Six Anatomical Tables*.[20] It is likely that multiple hands were involved in the preparation of the figures. According to the art historian Martin Kemp, the outlines of the muscle figures in *Fabrica* bear features from the Northern European tradition, and the landscapes in the background resemble the Venetian style of Domenico Campagnola, a painter as well as printmaker.[21] Campagnola was based in Padua while Vesalius was there, completing a set of monumental portraits of classical figures in the 'Hall of Giants' (1540).[22] Both Calcar and Campagnola are associated with Titian, though Titian himself was not involved in making the illustrations for *Fabrica*.[23]

In this period, those who designed or drew a composition did not usually cut the woodblocks. We do not know the identity of the cutters of the woodblocks either, though the interlocked capital letters I and O in the frontispiece (illus. 1) at the top to the left of the plaque might belong to one of them. The woodcuts in *Fabrica* are superb examples of the relief technique that skilfully translated the details of the original drawings. Compared to the woodcuts in Berengario's works, those in *Fabrica* are of superior quality, not only because the figures were larger (and therefore more details could be included), but also because of gradations and modelling achieved through hatching and cross-hatching of different density, as well as lines with softly tapering ends created by carving the end of lines with downward curves.[24] The suppleness of the lines and details of modelling were matched only by engraving techniques in the second half of the sixteenth century (illus. 74). We expect craftsmen of such singular skill to have been known in Venice to printers such as Francesco Marcolini who were publishing illustrated books, or to Titian and other artists expanding into the medium of woodcut.[25] The names of the woodcutters for *Fabrica* nevertheless remain elusive.

Though we do not know their names, we do know that Vesalius found that working with artists was not plain sailing, perhaps because of different expectations of what a human figure should look like. Vesalius remarked later that fretfulness of the artists made him feel unhappier than the cadavers that had landed on his dissection table.[26] Nevertheless, Vesalius was proud – as

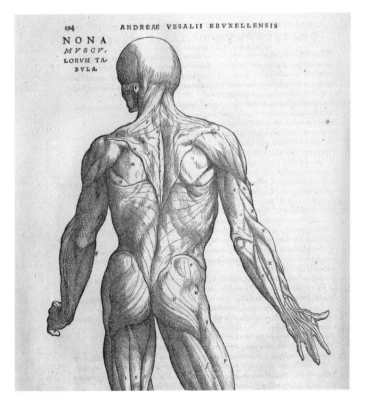

40 'An optical illusion, apparent . . . in the left arm, which is stretched forward and which someone ignorant of perspective might think was shorter than it should be.'

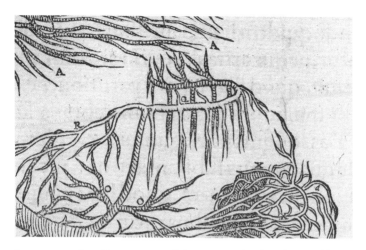

he expressed to Oporinus – of the 'pictorial rules' that had been applied to figures in *Fabrica*.[27] Vesalius did not expect his readers to be familiar with such rules, as he felt obliged to point out that 'someone ignorant of perspective' might think that the left arm in the ninth table of muscles (illus. 40) was shown as physically shorter than the right, rather than understanding that the arm was stretched forward (we now call this convention 'foreshortening').[28] Elsewhere, Vesalius specified the points of view from which the images were made – such as a cadaver lying on the ground or suspended upright (illus. 50).[29] He also thought it useful to explain the convention of modelling. At the vein marked Q (illus. 41) that followed the curvature of the stomach (*vena gastrica sinistra*), Vesalius explained that the blood vessels at the back had been shaded darker than those in the front and closer to view.[30] The black lines in the woodcuts were also used for indicating fibre directions and units of muscles, while the white spaces in between those lines did not by themselves indicate a structure. This convention mostly worked, except when Vesalius wanted to indicate the membranous structure in the middle of the abdomen (illus. 42), known as the 'white line' (*linea alba*). This structure was really white,

41 'The shading with which we have marked this vein [Q] . . . distinguished the part of the vein extending to the posterior and more hidden area from the part that is seen in the prior or anterior area, or is closer to the eyes.'

and Vesalius realized that its whiteness could not be shown without colouring in the fleshy parts, but he conceded that colouring all the figures would be expensive.[31] These comments indicate a clear appreciation on Vesalius's part of the visual conventions used in woodcuts.

What, if any, were the contributions of artists to *Fabrica*? It is tempting to believe that it was the draughtsman who chose the graceful pose of the muscle figures (illus. 38, 42) – one leg stepping forward with the weight of the body and the other leg at the back balancing the body – a pose mentioned by Alberti and adopted in earlier books on anatomy, now known as contrapposto (illus. 10, 17). The different angles of the leg meant that the calf muscle on the right leg (r in illus. 38) that was not fully visible on the other leg could be shown. The gesture in the second table of muscles (illus. 39) was noted many years ago by the art historian Erwin Panofsky as possibly resembling Titian's *Elocution of Alfonso d'Avalos* (1540).[32] Here again, the pose has the advantage of maximizing what can be included in one figure: namely, the muscles inside and outside the arms and legs. For similar reasons, the underside of the skull was also tilted slightly (illus. 43). Its advantage can be illustrated by comparing it to a woodcut (illus. 44) from the complete works of Galen (1538). The image in *Fabrica* loses the sense of symmetry evident in the 1538 woodcut, but it gains a view, on the right edge of the skull, of parts of the frontal bone, the coronal suture, the squamous conglutination, and the parietal bone. If these poses and positioning were the contribution of the artists who worked with Vesalius, they were also effective in maximizing their anatomical content.

Even with a tilt, it was not possible to show the whole of a three-dimensional body in one view. Leonardo showed the body from multiple angles, and Berengario used three. Just as he had done in his *Anatomical Tables*, Vesalius showed the bones in *Fabrica* from three angles. The first woodcut (illus. 45) shows an articulated

42 'R to X [in the centre of the body] shows a white line [*linea alba*], which it is not possible to express other than in a plain color. It would be worth the trouble to mark the illustrations in all copies with their own colors so that

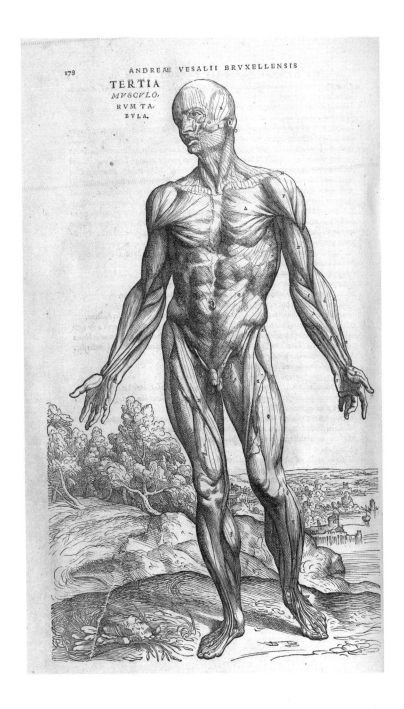

the membranous part could be most readily distinguished from the fleshy,
but for some the expense would be no small thing.'

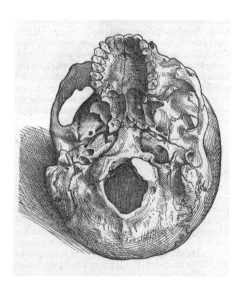
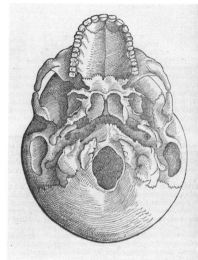

skeleton from the front resting its right arm on a shovel (a hint at gravedigging) so as to support the weight of the bones.[33] Vesalius noted that a 'skeleton', according to Galen, meant a set of bones joined up to form a 'dried cadaver'.[34]

The next figure, the skeleton in profile, with its legs crossed, leans on a classical sarcophagus, whose top has been tilted to show the skull it contemplates (illus. 46). This certainly improves on a similar composition in Berengario's book (illus. 18). *Fabrica*'s image is loosely based on prints by Dürer. The gesture of resting its head in its hand echoes the brooding figure of Dürer's 'Melencholia I' (1514), and the lines in Latin inscribed in italic capital letters on the side of the sarcophagus had been used in Dürer's engraving of his friend Willibald Pirckheimer (1524). The Latin inscription, in one translation, is rendered: 'Genius [*ingenio*] endures for aye; all the rest will pass away.'[35] At the time, it was believed to have been written by the Roman poet Virgil (first century BCE) on the death of his patron Maecenas, though (we now know) it could not have been by Virgil since he died before Maecenas. For Dürer,

43 Underside of the skull from *Fabrica* (1543).
44 Underside of the skull from Galen's *Works* (1538), shown upside down for comparison.

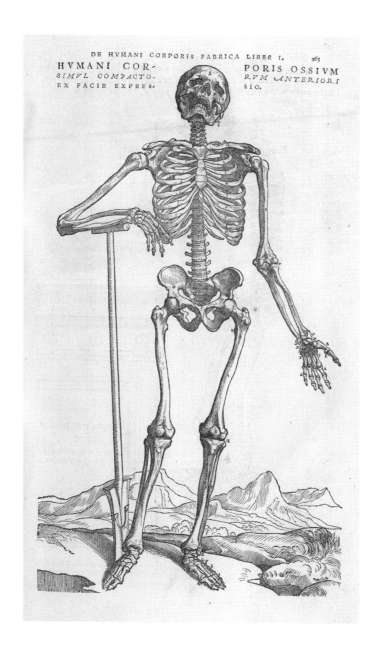

HVMANI COR-
*SIMVL COMPACTO-
EX FACIE EXPRES-*

PORIS OSSIVM
*RVM ANTERIORI
SIO.*

45 The arrangement of the bones depends 'on the nature of the stake
supporting the arms: one arrangement will suit a haymaker's scythe,
another a spear, and another a javelin or a Neptune's trident . . .'

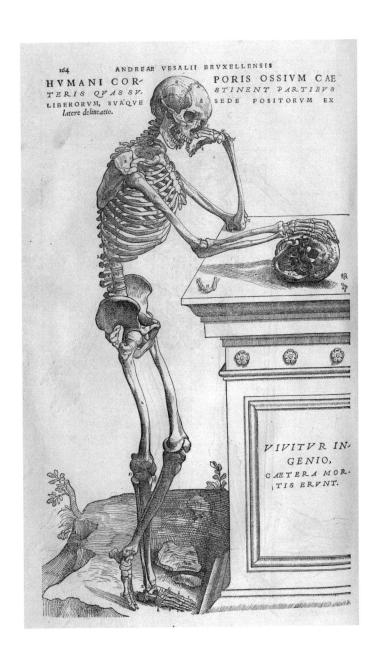

46 'Genius endures for aye; all the rest will pass away.'

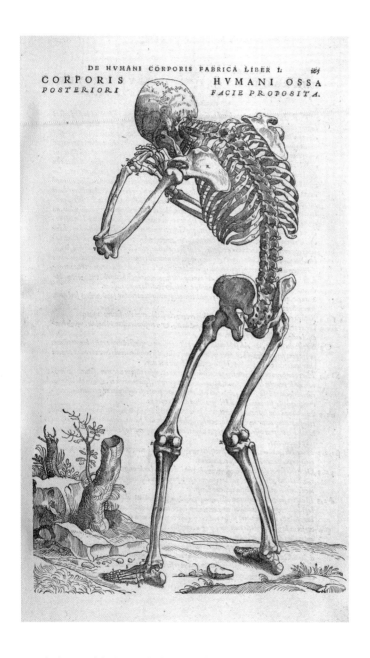

47 'The bones of the human body shown from the back.'

the lines conveyed the sense that he was only able to represent the features of his friend's physical body that would eventually perish, and not his immortal spirit.

Ingenium was not a word that Vesalius bandied about much. He used it in a general sense when singling out medicine as the most useful and difficult of all the arts to be discovered by human ingenuity.[36] When he cited Homer's approval of physicians and called the author of the *Iliad* the 'font of genius', he was repeating an epithet for Homer by Pliny the Elder.[37] Of his contemporaries, three were credited with possessing *ingenium* in the sense of talent: his compatriot and fellow student of medicine, Antonio Succha, was a 'young man of great talent'; Claudius Symionius was a law student 'of charm and talent'; and most importantly da Monte, the star professor who had recently arrived in Padua, was a man of 'the greatest, almost of divine genius'.[38] For Vesalius, the inscription on the side of the sarcophagus in *Fabrica* was not meant to signal any specific relationship with a patron or a friend, but it acknowledged the cultural link between a skeleton and death. When the woodcut was reused in *Epitome*, a different classical phrase was used with a more overt reference to death.[39]

In the third, posterior view (illus. 47), the skeleton bends its back so that its forehead almost touches its hands with interlocked fingers, a gesture of supplication. The three woodcuts on consecutive pages thus contained plenty of cues in their gestures, props and inscriptions to evoke the familiar trope of the ephemerality of life and the inevitability of death, a message that was not lost on contemporary readers or artists.[40] These images of skeletons in turn taught not only the names of the bones, but also how the bones enabled various poses and movements in life. Familiar imagery associated with death was thus pressed into the service of knowledge of the living human body.[41]

Another element that appears to be more decorative than anatomical, and thus could be considered an addition by artists, is the background of the muscle figures such as hilly landscapes with buildings or a hamlet, with the occasional obelisk, pyramid, aqueduct or arched ruin (illus. 38, 39, 42). These details are more finely rendered than those in the background to the muscle figures in Berengario's work (illus. 17). It is well known that the landscapes in *Fabrica* connect up to form two sequences – one sequence including all anterior views of the body and another of posterior views.[42] These sequential images may have been inspired by a popular imagery of the 'dance of death' – a procession of people from all walks of life being led to their grave by dancing skeletons. A mural depicting such a dance could be found at the Cemetery of Innocents at Paris which Vesalius frequented as a student. It was also a theme found in Hans Holbein the Younger's initials as well as his illustrations for episodes from the Old Testament.[43] A reader of *Fabrica* would not necessarily have noticed the artistic conceit of a continuous landscape, however, since the figures were not placed on consecutive pages. It nevertheless indicates that the ordering of the images was deliberate.

Vesalius said that he had a choice over the arrangement of the muscle figures: either all figures from the front could be shown first in the sequence of dissection followed by all figures from the back, or the anterior and the posterior views of the same stage of dissection could be shown alternately. His choice of the former, as confirmed by the continuous background, was essentially a preference for depth over three-dimensionality in the round. When looking at a muscle in one of the tables, his readers were told not to forget 'to look also at the preceding and following tables so as to discover what the muscle you are examining rests upon and what overlies it'.[44] The repeated contrapposto pose helped the reader identify the images as being layers of the same body (illus. 33, 38, 42).

One of the best-known artistic conceits in *Fabrica* is the use of the Belvedere Torso (illus. 48) to display the seminal vessels

and associated structures. This figure occurs towards the end
of a chapter on the viscera, where all the figures in that chapter
are of limbless torsos shown with the ends of the limbs shaded
like a stony surface rather than a cross section of a limb.[45] The
Belvedere Torso – without its arms and legs – was believed at the
time to represent the body of Hercules, which made for a good
prop to highlight Vesalius's earliest anatomical discoveries singled
out by Guenther: namely, that the seminal veins and arteries do
not initially run the same course.[46] The Belvedere Torso dignified
the anatomical structures placed in it as being as canonical and
heroic as a classical statue could be. It is also possible that it was
included in a deliberate one-upmanship over Berengario's figures
with sculptural references (illus. 17). Vesalius did not explicitly
mention the Torso in the text, but elsewhere he invoked the statues

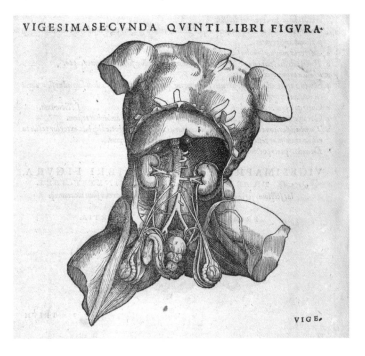

VIGESIMASECVNDA QVINTI LIBRI FIGVRA·

48 The Belvedere Torso in *Fabrica*; compare illus. 2.

'unearthed at Rome' to draw an analogy with the shape of a crown found in such a statue and the open state of the 'three-grooved process' (*valvula tricuspidalis*) of the heart.[47]

Vesalius was also careful about what to include in, or exclude from, an image. The muscle figures were all drawn from a cadaver suspended by a rope fixed to a pulley so that he could raise, lower or turn over the cadaver as required, which was important because if a body was left on the table, the muscles became stretched or compressed by the weight of the body and lost their natural form.[48] But this kind of support rope is visible only once in the muscle figures, in the seventh table, which helped to provide visual coherence to the contorted pose needed to show the inside of the ribcage (illus. 49). A clay brick placed under the neck to expose the throat was shown once, while some props which must have been used to show a scapula or a sacrum standing on its end were never mentioned or shown.[49] Some structures were not depicted at all because they were familiar – for example, the cartilage of the ear was essentially the same shape as the ear, so everyone knew how it looked. Other structures like ligaments that covered the bones could not be drawn separately, and readers were urged to imagine their shape from the outline of the bones. And the various curves and curls of the nerves 'most delightful to the sight' were beyond depiction and best appreciated in a dissection.[50]

On one occasion, Vesalius explained why he decided not to include a particular drawing. This was a drawing of the corpus callosum in the brain held up with two hands so as to show the septum (*septum pellucidum*) underneath it intact.[51] Vesalius decided the drawing did not work as well as it did in an actual dissection, and was not worth wasting space. Avoiding waste of space was often cited as a reason for not including or repeating illustrations – though it was also the case that a couple of woodcuts (showing a large number of details) were printed twice to illustrate different anatomical details.[52] The implication was that unnecessary use

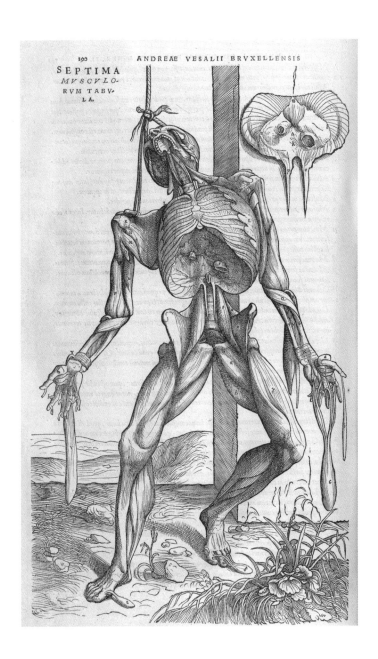

SEPTIMA
MVSCVLO-
RVM TABV-
LA.

49 'This is how the cadaver was suspended for drawing all the muscle tables.'

of paper would increase unjustifiably the cost of production and thus the price of the book. Explaining that he was not overindulgent in his use of images meant that the cost of the book was justified. The cancelled drawing would also have been the only image to have shown the hands of a dissector.

The human figure could be beautiful, and it could be informative. Artists believed in the benefits of being familiar with human anatomy, but this was ultimately subservient to their idea of beauty and artistic expression. Authors of anatomical tracts relied on these artists to convey information on human anatomy. Each hoped that their human figures would be convincing to their audience. For Berengario the art enthusiast, the inclusion of a well-known sculpture or pictorial motif was about displaying the connoisseurial taste that he shared with his noble patrons. They made little difference to his discussion of the anatomical structure of the body. Vesalius sought to harness artists' skill to convey anatomical information efficiently and effectively. The images of *Fabrica* were just as carefully staged and constructed as any other artwork, and the bodies were not always shown in their 'natural position', as Vesalius himself acknowledged.[53] What is unusual in the case of Vesalius as an author is the extent to which he was visually aware, and actively directed how the figures should look and what should be included or omitted. He must have believed in the power of images to create anatomical knowledge.

SIX

Theatre

abrica's frontispiece showed spectators lining a tiered, wooden scaffold curved around a central table. It showed, as Vesalius said, half of the kind of theatre prepared for him in Padua and Bologna.[1] Theatres where public anatomies took place were not yet purpose-built spaces, however. When Vesalius visited Bologna, his dissections took place in the Church of St Francis where the medical faculty elected its rector. There, a table and four steps of benches were installed 'so that nearly 200 persons could see the anatomy'.[2]

At the time, churches were the most commonly available roofed spaces large enough for sizeable gatherings. Vesalius's doctoral examination took place in the Church of St Urban in Padua, and his degree ceremony was held in the palace of the Bishop of Padua.[3] Other spaces used in Padua included the hall of the hospital of St Francis for examination for law degrees, and the apothecary's shop at the sign of the Lamb of God for smaller meetings of the faculty of arts and medicine.[4] We do not know for certain, however, where Vesalius's lectures or anatomies took place in Padua.[5] There was no classical building corresponding to the one in the frontispiece while Vesalius was there. Wherever it was, mounting a public anatomy involved complex arrangements. Contrary to the impression of the frontispiece – that there is a single protagonist in the whole of the theatre – a number of people had to be involved for such a public anatomy to happen at all.

JUDICIAL AUTHORITIES

As Heseler complained, the year before Vesalius visited Bologna, the rector of the medical faculty had not bothered to ask for a body of an executed criminal since he was not interested in anatomy.[6] Even if the rector was willing to make the request, agreement from judicial powers was also needed to obtain bodies of the executed. This was a statutory stipulation set up earlier to avoid the suspicion that bodies had been obtained illicitly.

The highest judicial authority in Padua was the *podestà*, a position occupied by a member of the Venetian Senate for one or two years at a time. Between 1539 and 1541, Marcantonio Contarini of the well-known Venetian patrician family served as *podestà*.[7] Contarini, praised by Vesalius as 'renowned throughout the world for his peerless knowledge of philosophy and languages and for so many ambassadorial missions completed with brilliant success', was also thanked for the 'plentiful' supply of bodies. Vesalius added that Contarini was a most 'attentive and tireless observer of the fabric of the human body', like another Flavius Boethius or Sergius Paulus, the two Roman consuls mentioned by Galen in *On Anatomical Procedures*.[8] Galen's political supporters were knowledgeable about anatomy – so were Vesalius's. Thus, the burgomaster of Louvain, Adriaan van Blehen, who was 'glad to grant' Vesalius any corpse, was lauded for 'no ordinary knowledge of anatomy' and for eagerly attending his anatomies.[9] Vesalius flattered his political supporters as being as knowledgeable as the ancient Roman elites, which implied that anatomical knowledge was valued beyond the medical profession.

The criminal justice system in pre-modern Europe meted out various forms of corporal punishment such as removal of eyes, tongues, ears or hands, and executions by hanging, decapitation, drowning, breaking on a wheel or quartering.[10] Several of these required cutting into the criminal's body. Vesalius mentioned that cutting the tendon of the 'fifth muscle moving the foot [*musculus*

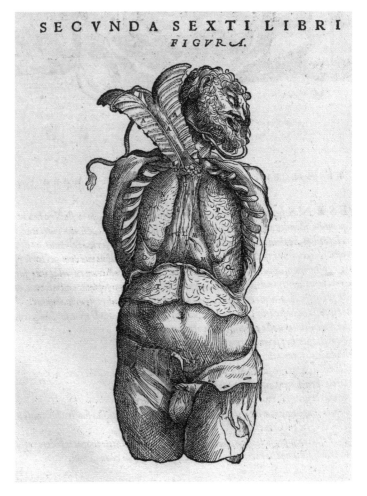

SECVNDA SEXTI LIBRI
FIGVRA.

tibialis posterior]' was the worst punishment that could be inflicted on a person next to death, though he was not advocating it as a form of punishment.[11] It is unlikely that Vesalius assisted in punishments of criminals. These were usually undertaken by public executioners, who often had a parallel career in healing based on their familiarity with the human body.[12] Vesalius noted how a

50 'This figure is erect, not lying down.' A remnant of a noose holds up the breast bones.

youth hanged in Padua whose body was made available for public anatomy had had his right eye gouged out a year earlier by an executioner.[13] Vesalius was also a bystander rather than a participant at an execution where the heart had been taken out of a living person at Bologna. In a similar instance in Padua, he managed to examine the 'still beating' heart, lung and viscera of a person who had been quartered alive at a pharmacist's shop near the place of execution.[14] Though the historian Andrea Carlino found a case in Rome in 1587 where the punishment of quartering was replaced with a public anatomy at the Sapienza University, it was rare for a public anatomy to substitute for criminal punishment.[15]

The manner of execution also had implications for the subsequent anatomy. Vesalius remarked that strangulation by a noose made it difficult to take the skin off the compressed area of the neck.[16] On one occasion (illus. 50), a noose around the neck was shown in *Fabrica*'s woodcut as a prop to hold up the sternum with rib cartilages in an erect figure to show its interior surface as well as the thorax.[17] This is a rare instance where an image hints at a (still partially clothed) criminal's body.

Even if the *podestà* was favourably inclined, not every executed body could be released for public anatomies. The statutes of the University of Padua prohibited the use of the bodies of a citizen of Venice or Padua, of a member of a local family of distinction or of a foreign nobleman. In Bologna, bodies had to be of a person who came from at least 30 miles away. These conditions were probably meant to avoid recognition of the body and shame on the family of the executed.[18]

Yet, a citizen of Padua who was imprisoned for three years until he died of black jaundice was a subject of Vesalius's public anatomy.[19] If a body could not be located within Padua, the statutes urged the rector to find one from nearby Venice or elsewhere in the Paduan territories. This was probably the reason why one of the bodies in Vesalius's public anatomy came from Monticelli

Terme, about 140 kilometres (87 mi.) southwest of Padua. Intriguingly, this man was not completely unknown in Venice or Padua either:

> He had been a youth with an extremely white and hairless skin, and not at all melancholic by nature. He was so popular for his Diogenic way of life that he three times escaped the noose. The first time, he was flogged in Venice, and then came to Padua, where he was punished with the removal of his right eye and hand. After being arrested a second time in Montiselli (he had broken out of prison there once already), he played out the final act of his tragedy.[20]

Career criminals were often known for their deeds or escapades, some of which could even strike a chord with the public. This was likely the case here as Diogenes was a classical figure noted for scorning material possessions and denouncing wealth, power and corruption. The university's stipulations were not meant to exclude bodies such as this Diogenic thief's cadaver because he could be recognized. In practice, local recognition of the body was not an overriding factor in withholding corpses for a public anatomy unless they were members of distinguished families.

Other bodies of the executed that Vesalius mentioned in *Fabrica* belonged to a beautiful prostitute who had been hung in Paris, a young woman with only one functioning eye hung in Padua, a man whose 'warm' head Vesalius was able to inspect less than quarter of an hour after his beheading, a woman who tried to avoid execution by falsely claiming pregnancy, and possibly an oarsman of a papal boat.[21] Bodies of executed criminals were not abundant. The historian Paul Grendler noted that Venice executed nine individuals between 1520 and 1569, in comparison to 22 in the preceding 20 years.[22] We do not have the corresponding number of executions for Padua, about a quarter of the size of Venice.[23] In practice, bodies for public anatomies had to be supplemented from elsewhere, such as local hospitals where someone destitute or without family had died. Those who had not died at the hands of the executioner and whose bodies Vesalius had dissected included a workman who had accidentally fallen off a ladder at a quarry, a French priest who died 'of water under the skin' at a hostel in Bologna, a prostitute who hanged herself in Padua, a woman who was killed by her husband with a cudgel, and a man who had died of inflammation of the brain.[24] In these cases, presumably some permission had been given by the families of the deceased, or by those in charge of hostels in the case of travellers, though it is not clear that these bodies were dissected publicly.

Two female bodies were delivered to Vesalius's public anatomies by students.[25] One was the body of the mistress of a monk of the Church of St Anthony who had died of a 'strangulation of the womb or a stroke' and the other of a 'very old little woman' who died of starvation during the famine of 1539–40. These are, in fact, the rare instances where Vesalius mentioned who had brought the body to the theatre. Both bodies had been stolen from their graves by students. The family of the monk's mistress complained to the *podestà*. Such grave robbings must have happened often enough for the Paduan authorities to feel the need to prohibit it explicitly in 1547.[26]

STUDENT ORGANIZERS

The arrangement of a public anatomy at Padua and Bologna normally fell on two medical students elected as *masarii* (meaning mace-bearers in Latin) who had been medical students for at least two years and had preferably seen an anatomy before.[27] Their task was to prepare a place for the public anatomy, provide instruments and all other necessary things for the dissection, and collect fees from those attending so as to cover the cost of the event, usually assisted by the university beadle who was in charge of gatherings, records and fees.

We do not know the details of the tasks of these student organizers at Padua or Bologna in this period, but we can catch a glimpse of what might have been involved from the University of Montpellier. From the financial records of the equivalent student officers (called 'procurators') at Montpellier, we know that materials used in a public anatomy of a woman who had died in a hospital in 1527 included candles, incense (to ameliorate the stench from the cadaver), sponges, towels and cloths for the dissector to wipe their hands, wood and coal for the fire in the dissection room, and a glass vase to store the intestines.[28] Payments were made to the custodian of the hospital and his wife, the porters who carried the body from the hospital to the university, the university beadle for opening the doors and preparing the room for the anatomy, his wife for cleaning the room, and his sons for fetching items during the dissection. All this came to just over two livres. Jean Falcon, one of the royal professors of medicine, described by the student procurator as the 'very splendid and singular interpreter of the history of the body', was paid three livres and the dissector one livre. The total cost of the anatomy thus came to just over six livres. The funeral, however, cost twice as much. The priests, a plot in the cemetery, the gravediggers, the paupers forming the funeral cortège, the coffin and the Mass for the soul of the deceased came to twelve livres. Organizing all of this was quite a challenge – the two student procurators reported that they felt overwhelmed by the countless tasks involved in preparing a public anatomy across three days and in organizing the funeral. All of which they believed justified a remuneration of just over half a livre to themselves.

It appears that there was no formal arrangement between the hospital and the university. On this occasion, 'a poor little woman' had informed the procurator that a woman had just died in the hospital whom the university might want for dissection. The student procurator tipped her 12 deniers (which would buy 2 pounds of candle wax at the time). He also gave a gratuity to the wife of the hospital custodian, 'so that she may be favourably disposed to let the procurator know when cadavers appropriate for dissection might become available next'. Student organizers needed to cultivate local contacts and informants in order to procure a body.

Schedel had noted that the body for the public anatomy was buried with great pomp, and the example from Montpellier above confirms that it was common practice to pay for the funeral of those who were dissected at a public anatomy. This was also the

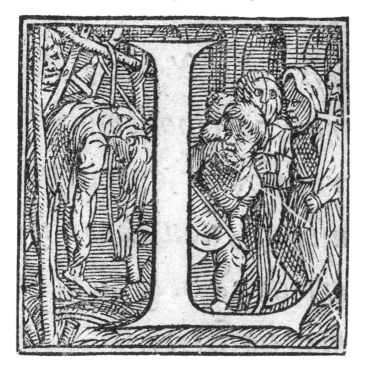

51 A hanged criminal lowered from the gallows while a priest and a member of a confraternity look on. Woodcut 3.7 centimetres/1½ in. square.

case even with executed criminals, who were looked after in their final days by religious groups. In Bologna, the confraternity of St Mary of Death (Santa Maria della Morte) formalized from October 1541 what appears to have been a pre-existing custom of providing a body for anatomy to the university on condition that the professor paid in advance for the Mass for the executed.[29] The stipulation 'in advance' suggests that there had earlier been problems with the payment for the Mass.

The background of the initial L in *Fabrica* shows a body of a hung criminal being lowered from the gallows, with a priest holding a cross next to a member of a confraternity whose identity is protected with a hood covering the face (illus. 51).[30] This indicates the legitimate means by which bodies were acquired, in

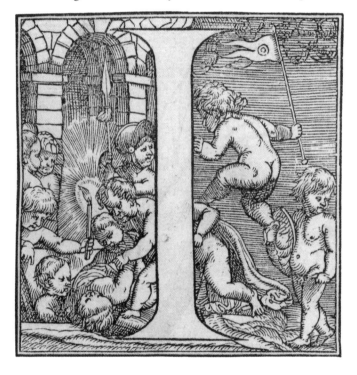

52 Putti digging up a body under candlelight. 7.5 centimetres/3 in. square.

contrast to the grave robbing perpetrated by putti by candlelight visible in the background to the initial I (illus. 52). The putti may well be a reference to medical students.[31]

In *Fabrica*, Vesalius did not explicitly mention any student organizers, but there are scattered references to those whose help he relied upon in his public anatomies. He always had a porter present when the intestines needed to be cleaned out, who may have helped also with washing and preparing the body for dissection. In his public anatomies, the additional pair of hands of an attendant was sometimes needed – to lift the stomach in order to show the origin of the lower membrane of the omentum, for instance.[32] These attendants were probably servants rather than the student organizers or other students.

SPECTATORS

A public anatomy would not be public without its spectators. We do not, however, have a record of the precise numbers of those attending anatomies, let alone of those attending the university. The total number of students in the 1530s at Padua is estimated at around 1,100.[33] If we assume that the proportion of the number of medical degrees awarded to the total number of degrees conferred in the same year (an average of about 15 per cent between 1536 and 1540) is reflected in the overall student numbers, the number of students pursuing a medical degree would have been about 160 to 170 students a year, with the remainder being mostly students of law.[34]

Even though the faculty of medicine at Bologna was larger than that at Padua, we should probably treat with caution Berengario da Carpi's claim that nearly five hundred students and citizens were present at his anatomy, not least because of the practicality of accommodating so many people in a single space.[35] 'Five hundred' may have been a way to express an impressively large number. On the other hand, when Heseler reported that more than 150 students were present at Vesalius's anatomy at Bologna in 1540, it sounds plausible, though attendance may have been higher than usual because of a guest lecturer from Padua.[36] The fact that in the second edition of *Fabrica* Vesalius stated that a theatre should be able to hold 'fifty or more' indicates a lower threshold, and it is possible that the number of spectators fluctuated significantly.[37] Even if we cannot determine the actual number of those who attended public anatomies, it is certainly the case that the Bolognese rules from the early fifteenth century capping the maximum number of students at twenty for an anatomy of a male body and thirty for a female body were honoured in the breach by this time.[38]

Heseler noted that there were about 200 spectators – of whom about 150 were students – at the start of Vesalius's anatomy at Bologna in 1540. Those other than students who could attend a public anatomy were the rector and his guest, professors of the university, and any member of the local college of physicians.[39] In practice, the composition of the audience seemed to change depending on the topic of the dissection. Heseler noted that some of the professors left when Vesalius turned to the anatomy of muscles. When it came to the topic of the organs of generation, many theologians turned up. According to Vesalius, judges and mayors also attended his anatomies. Though possibly included in *Fabrica*'s frontispiece, Vesalius never mentioned that women were in his audience.

Benedetti's imaginary public dissections were attended by the political and intellectual elites after the medical students had left the theatre. Berengario stated that Bolognese citizens were among the audience of his public anatomies. Massa cited his learned Venetian peers as witnesses to his discoveries. A non-medical, elite presence at public anatomies furthermore opened up the possibility of the anatomical theatre becoming a place

where anatomical facts could be endorsed and authenticated
by others with high status. Vesalius followed his predecessors in
citing spectators as witnesses: 'nobody in the whole assemblage
of learned men was able to deny' the course of the azygos vein.[40]
When Vesalius proudly declared that everything in *Fabrica* had
been demonstrated in his public anatomies in Padua and Bologna,
he was implying endorsement by the spectators.[41]

For all the preparations that went into mounting a public
dissection, Vesalius found his main audience – the students –
disappointingly inattentive. This was probably because he was
straying from the traditional, Mondinian focus on the major
organs in the three venters that left the discussion of muscles,
bones and blood vessels to the very end. Following Galen's *On
Anatomical Procedures*, Vesalius inverted this order and began with
the bones and muscles. Heseler – who had already attended a
dissection of a thief when studying medicine at Leipzig, probably
in the Mondinian manner – barely made notes about the bones
with which Vesalius began. Again, when Vesalius insisted on
describing the muscles at length, Heseler's sympathy was more
with the professors who had left the theatre – he felt that knowledge of muscles was more necessary for surgeons than for physicians, but he decided to stay on, as he thought it useful to have
seen them 'once'.[42]

There was certainly a gap between what Vesalius was doing
and what students were expecting. Students at Bologna thought
that his comment that anyone can see the anatomical structure
themselves was a sign of ambition and disrespect for authorities.[43]
When at the end of the anatomy the students asked for the 'truth'
of an anatomical matter, Vesalius replied that he did not want
to give his own opinion because he wanted them to find out for
themselves. 'Feel with your own hands and trust them,' he urged.
This reply was greeted with dismay. The students saw it as Vesalius
jealously guarding his views (*invidum*), and unwilling to share them

with others. Inculcating a new attitude of first-hand dissection turned out to be difficult, as students preferred to be told what was correct rather than finding things out for themselves.

There was further predictable student behaviour: some were more interested in being able to impress their peers by boasting that 'forty' muscles were demonstrated in the anatomy without taking any detailed notes, or they complained that Vesalius covered 'far too much in a single demonstration'.[44] Others who wanted to appear more studious took down notes focusing on where Vesalius disagreed with Galen, but they often missed the point. The 'negligence of the spectators' brought home to Vesalius the difficulty of getting students to grasp his points in public anatomies. They were noisy and unruly, which made Vesalius flustered and angry.[45] The theatre was perhaps not the best place to teach human anatomy to students after all.

THE CONDUCT OF PUBLIC ANATOMY

We only have sporadic information on the actual procedures of public anatomies regarding the time of the year, frequency, duration or the manner in which they were conducted. Both Bologna and Padua expected at least one public anatomy of a male cadaver and, where possible, one of a female body each year, during the winter months. Vesalius confirmed in *Fabrica* that bodies of a male and a female were dissected in a public anatomy in Padua in one year.[46] It may have been less frequent than Montpellier, which held 29 public anatomies between 1526 and 1535.[47]

Public anatomies were expected to take place during the winter months when the cadaver putrefied more slowly than in the warmer season. There was, however, no stipulation about the duration of the dissection as it probably depended on the condition of the body available. Giovanni Antonio Lonigo's anatomy in Padua lasted for a month from 24 December 1536 to 24 January

1537; Vesalius's first public anatomy in Padua took place from 6 to 24 December in 1537 and his dissection in Bologna from 15 to 29 January 1540; Schedel attended a public anatomy that lasted five days in March.[48] Vesalius's dissection in Basle of Jacob Karrer, a bigamist who attacked his first wife and left her for dead, was in May. But this was an impromptu event that took advantage of an execution while he was overseeing the publication of his book, as the local university did not have a tradition of regular public anatomies.[49]

More often than not, a public anatomy was conducted with a single cadaver. Following Galen, Vesalius recommended that public anatomies should start with the bones as the basic structure of the body; he thus brought an articulated skeleton with him. As if to invite his audience to 'see through' to the bones inside the body, he drew outlines of the bones on the skin, and then explained how the names of the parts of the body were taken from names of the bones.[50] The nude figures in *Epitome* surrounded by the names of the parts of the body (illus. 53) hint at this stage of the anatomy before dissection. After this, Vesalius recommended the examination of the organs in the abdominal cavity, followed by those in the thoracic area.[51] One side of the body was used for dissecting the muscles moving the arm, the scapula, the thorax, the back and the head; the other side for blood vessels and nerves. The brain was to be dissected next, followed by the muscles moving the forearm, wrist and fingers, then those moving the lower leg, thigh, foot and toes, and finally the veins, arteries and nerves in the arm and leg. Some of the structures were difficult to see: Vesalius made students leave the hall and come back in groups so that they could take turns in seeing the course of the bile duct, for example.[52] He also used images from his *Anatomical Tables* or drew with charcoal on the dissecting table to show the course of veins, arteries and nerves.[53] What he could show in a public anatomy depended on the state of the body, but he also adjusted what to include depending on the 'expertise of the spectators'.[54]

The use of just one cadaver for a public anatomy presented certain limitations. Some structures could be damaged (for example, because of the manner of execution) or difficult to examine (perhaps because of too much fat), or some parts had to be destroyed in order to reach other parts. To compensate for this, Vesalius recommended the use of animals. General structures of bones, cartilages, fat, tendons and so on could be shown in a dog or a lamb without wasting the human body; kidneys of dogs were easier to examine than those in a fat human; and a clearer idea of the structure of the larynx could be obtained by dissecting ones from an ox or a calf before dissecting one in the human body. Parts from animal bodies thus supplemented a single-body dissection.[55]

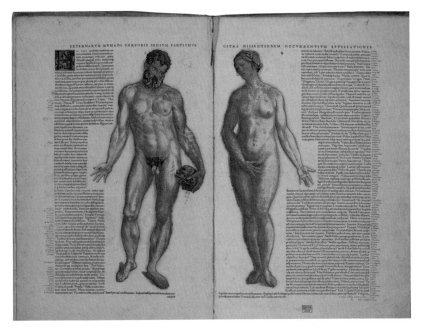

53 The yet-to-be-dissected male and female figures in *Epitome* (1543), surrounded by the names of the parts of the body, with the Greek names in the margin.

By the time Vesalius conducted his guest demonstrations in Bologna, the senior professor was no longer present in the theatre to read out or comment on Mondino's text.[56] Matteo Corti, Bologna's senior professor and the foremost Galenist of his time, gave his lectures separately from the anatomy. For Corti, anatomy consisted of the art of dissection by deed (actual dissection that determined the position, shape, size and quantity of parts of the body) and by word (description that explained the functions of those parts).[57] He considered the latter the purview of philosophers and physicians. His aim was to replace Mondino's descriptions with Galen's. This necessitated lengthy and extensive commentary on the various works of Galen, which were weighed up against views of other classical authorities. Corti therefore needed a separate series of lectures.

This separation meant that it was relatively easy for Vesalius to take control of the proceedings in the theatre. Corti and the other professors of medicine attended his public anatomy sometimes, but not always. Vesalius effectively took over what used to be the senior professors' task of reading out and commenting on the text – he cited or summarized Galen's views.[58] He then introduced his own views that were contrary to the views of Galen – and of Corti too.

A war of words erupted. On entering the theatre, Vesalius declared that 'we must leave Galen and look at the body.'[59] Corti replied no, 'we must not leave Galen because he always well understood everything, and consequently we will follow him.' Vesalius proceeded to show the course of azygos veins that had implications for the appropriate bloodletting points for the affliction known as 'pain of the side'. He had published his views on the affliction, but so had Corti, three times. Corti replied that there might be other kinds of vessels. Vesalius demanded that he be shown in the body where such vessels were, since he dealt with things that were manifest, not hidden. Corti retorted, 'I am no anatomist.' He said that he dealt with things that were very evident to the mind. With mild condescension, he added that Vesalius did not know the works of Hippocrates or Galen terribly well. Vesalius bristled at this suggestion. The clash was ultimately about status and authority. Corti dismissed out of hand Vesalius's claims because Vesalius did not have the requisite authority or learning to disagree with Galen – or himself. This clash in the theatre, Heseler observed, 'accomplished nothing'.

The experience in Bologna must have spurred Vesalius in his resolve to write another book, which was completed by the summer of 1542. The theatre – the place of public anatomies – was an important arena for Vesalius to establish his authority by winning over spectators. It could serve as a forum for social and collective authentication. But in order to win an argument over the likes of Corti, Vesalius knew that he had to make a move from the theatre back to a book.

SEVEN

The Bodies in the Book

n moving from the theatre to the book, Vesalius retained a close link to the theatre, and not just in the frontispiece. The content of *Fabrica* was arranged to follow the order of his public anatomies. It thus started with the bones and cartilages, followed by muscles and ligaments, moving on to the veins, arteries and nerves, and then to the organs in the abdomen, thorax and finally the brain.[1] As we have just seen, a variety of bodies ended up on Vesalius's dissection table – those who had met their death naturally, accidentally, violently or by the executioner. However, *Fabrica* was not set up as a series of reports from the theatre about his individual dissections.

The advantage of a book was that Vesalius could describe his view of the human body more fully and defend it in more detail than time or a single cadaver might allow in a public anatomy. More importantly, Vesalius could collate observations from different bodies made at different times and extrapolate from them. Anatomical knowledge was not just about this or that particular body, but about a more general body which did not have the idiosyncrasies of an individual dissected in the theatre. Bodies other than the ones he had dissected were included in *Fabrica* in order to establish a general knowledge about the human body. They are the focus of this chapter.

CANONICAL AND INDIVIDUAL BODIES

While Vesalius acknowledged that in a private anatomy any type of body would be acceptable, it was desirable in a public anatomy to use one that was not 'monstrous'. Benedetti had recommended a body that was of middle age, not too thin, not too fat. Vesalius also emphasized the desirability of a middle-aged body that had a well-balanced temperament (the physical constitution arising from the combination of the four humours) proper to its sex. However, he was hardly in a position to pick such a suitable body from an abundance of cadavers. What this meant in practice was that Vesalius had to ignore idiosyncrasies of an individual body encountered in the theatre.[2] He would skip over uncommon features in case students thought they existed in all bodies. In a public anatomy, students would have been ill-served by a cadaver that was markedly different from what Vesalius called a 'canon' of the human body.

'Canon' is how Vesalius expressed what we today may call a normal or average body, but 'normal' and 'average' were not quite the words used by him. Vesalius drew on a classical idea derived from the work of a renowned sculptor in ancient Greece, Polycleitus (active c. 450–420 BCE). His sculpture was called the canon, which in turn achieved 'canonical' status because later sculptors came to compare their own work against it.[3] Vesalius likened the body most suitable for a public dissection to Polycleitus' statue against which other bodies could be compared.

Vesalius was not the first to associate Polycleitus' canon with a human body. Galen had used 'canon' to express a human body whose parts were perfectly well proportioned in relation to each other and embodied perfection of every type of humoral balance, though he doubted whether such a perfection would be found in a single individual. Such a canonical human body was the object of study in *Fabrica*. This meant that 'unnatural monstrosities' such as hermaphrodites were excluded from his discussion.[4] Also ruled out of the book were the bodies of Christ and of Adam. When discussing the bloating of the body in executed criminals left in the sun, Vesalius pointed out that this description should not be used in explaining the blood and water that issued from the side of the body of Christ when a soldier pierced him on the cross.[5] Furthermore, if Adam's skeleton had been articulated, it would have had one fewer rib (as it was used to create Eve), but that did not mean that all men lacked a rib.[6] The bodies of Christ and of Adam were thus omitted from consideration in *Fabrica* because inference from the human body did not apply to the former and inference from the latter could not be applied to humans.

Public anatomies carried the risk of extrapolating from a single cadaver with too many deviations from the canonical body. To counter this, frequent dissection was needed, just as Galen had urged students to dissect as many human bodies as possible before challenging him. Yet a canonical body did not exactly equate to an aggregate of dissected bodies. Vesalius – as with earlier writers on anatomy – considered anatomy a part of natural philosophy. This meant identifying a 'purpose' for each part of the body. 'Purpose' was important in Aristotelian philosophy, which was also adopted by Galen: parts of the body were shaped and structured in a particular way so as to fulfil certain functions.[7] It explained how the body was made.

Vesalius's commitment to making anatomy philosophical meant that consideration of function sometimes overrode frequency of occurrence of a feature. As noted by Straus and Temkin, a rare ossicle found underneath the little finger (N in illus. 54) in the hand (it is also present in the foot) is found in 0.1 per cent of Caucasians. It was included in *Fabrica*'s canonical body because Vesalius found a function for it: to stop the little finger from slipping down.[8] Vesalius also considered canonical a small foramen in the skull occasionally seen on one side of the sphenoid bone (and even more rarely on both sides), because it transmitted a

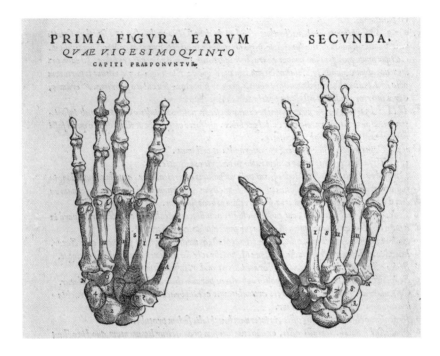

PRIMA FIGVRA EARVM   SECVNDA.
QV AE V.IGESIMOQVINTO
CAPITI PRAEPONVNTVR.

vein that connected the inside and outside of the skull (S in
illus. 43). Vesalius thus described the human body using the
classically inspired idea of an ideal body (canon) and a similarly
classical idea of function (purpose). Anatomical knowledge
explained why the human body was made in the way that it was.

It turns out that it is the rare variants that now bear his name.
The ossicle in the bone of the hand (or toe) was named *os Vesalianum
carpi* (or *tarsi*) in the nineteenth century. In the aftermath of Charles
Darwin's work on evolution, anatomists began reviewing historical works on anatomy for recorded cases of variations in the
human body which they believed could be clues to human development. Wilhelm Pfitzner, based at a new anatomical institute
at Strasbourg for anatomy, palaeontology and developmental
history, noted that the ossicle at the bottom of the little finger

54 N: 'This bone, when present, seems to strengthen the joint and give some
support to the metacarpal bone which sustains the little finger.'

described by Vesalius had not been observed again until 1870 by
Wenzel Gruber, professor of anatomy at the Medical Academy
of St Petersburg. In honour of its first discoverer, Pfitzner named
the ossicle after Vesalius.[9] It is less clear who named the foramen
in the sphenoid bone after Vesalius.[10] The 'foramen of Vesalius'
was also a structure that received attention in the nineteenth century by those interested in variation and comparative anatomy.
Alexander Macalister, the second holder of the chair of anatomy
at the University of Cambridge, established its existence in the
minke whale, and included it in his *Text-Book of Human Anatomy*
(1889), noting that it could sometimes be absent.[11] Macalister owned
a copy of *Epitome* (illus. 3) as well as a copy of *Fabrica* given to him
by Sir Hugh Kerr Anderson, another physiologist interested in
variation.

Vesalius's focus on the canonical body did not mean that he
ignored variation altogether or that the canonical body was rigidly
fixed in shape and structure. Of the five skulls shown in *Fabrica*
(illus. 55), only the top left figure marked 'first' (*prima*) was defined
as 'natural'.[12] The other four deviations from it were described as
'not natural', though modern anatomists would regard all of them
as within the range of normal variation rather than pathological.
In *Fabrica*, the 'natural' figure of a skull was described as the shape
of a sphere, elongated along its front and the back. Variation from
this shape was listed systematically – skulls lacking the anterior
prominence only (second figure), the posterior prominence only
(third figure) and both prominences (fourth figure), and cases
where the skull was broader to the sides than the length from the
back to the front (fifth figure). These shapes had been listed in
Hippocrates' *Head Wounds*. Vesalius took the opportunity to make
a learned reference from Homer's *Iliad* to the ugliest man in the
Greek army, Thersites, whose misshapen head was an example
of the fourth figure. As for the fifth shape, Galen had said that
while theoretically possible, it could not occur in nature. Vesalius

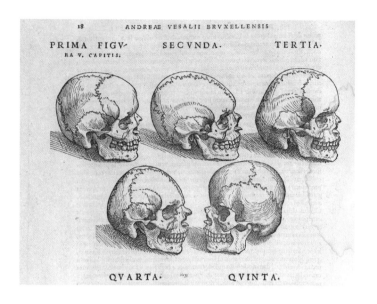

immediately added that he had seen a child in Venice with such a head who was also deformed in other parts of the body and was mentally deficient. In other words, Vesalius was showing that he knew all the possible skull shapes discussed by ancient authors and introduced his own experience to show Galen's lack of it. He added further shapes he had seen – a squarish head of a beggar in Bologna, and a child with a head larger than two natural heads who was shown around door-to-door by a beggar woman in Genoa. These expanded the range of shapes that diverged from the 'natural' shape. However, Vesalius did not directly link skull shapes deviating from the 'natural' one with mental defects, as he knew extremely intelligent people who had 'unnatural' head shapes.[13]

Not all deviations from the canon were 'monstrous'. The ability to move one's ears was not a mark of stupidity, as Vesalius pointed out in the case of a Paduan friend, Claudius Symionius of Friuli, who had recently obtained a doctorate in both canon and civil law.[14] Another acquaintance, Joannes Centurio of Genoa,

55 'All shapes varying from [the first one] are considered not natural.'

was cited as an example (the Latin word Vesalius used was *specimen*) of looseness of finger joints: he had long and elegant fingers which could be bent backwards to hold water as could be done in the palm. As if to emphasize the fact that there was nothing freakish about such a case, Vesalius added that Centurio (probably a member of the prestigious Genoese clan) was 'a young man of great promise and precise judgement and outstanding alike in the nobility of his family, the integrity of his conduct, and his remarkable knowledge of good literature and other disciplines'.[15] Just as Benedetti or Massa had mentioned their friends and colleagues in their books, Vesalius made a point of citing his acquaintances by name. The bodies of intellectually and socially respectable individuals who were personally known to Vesalius contributed to the reliability of the anatomical knowledge presented in *Fabrica*.

Variation was also highlighted by the bodies of the Turks. Turks had been a regular presence in Venice because of trading links (notwithstanding frequent skirmishes) with the Mamluks and subsequently the Ottomans. In the Western European imagination, the 'Turks' were an object of fear and fascination for their military prowess and their distinctive cultural traditions.[16] Vesalius typified this attitude when he cited Turks who were stronger in physique than Europeans. The potential strength of the temporal muscle was illustrated by a Turkish performer at Padua who had hurled with his teeth an 11-kilogram (25-lb) iron spike from the ground into a wall behind him which was 12 metres (39 ft) away – Vesalius had measured the distance himself.[17] A more impressive example from hearsay was that of a Turkish man in Venice who could easily pick up with his teeth a log that took five men to lift. It was not that the Turks had different anatomical structures, but that they had developed stronger muscles. A range of individual bodies was cited in *Fabrica* to enable Vesalius to illustrate different types of variation.

Ordinary, unnamed people going about their own business were also invoked in *Fabrica* to illustrate the workings of the canonical body. The fact that the lower leg could flex or extend only vertically when the thigh was motionless could be seen when people used their feet to 'soften leather on wooden platforms or when bakers in many countries knead the dough by treading on it', and the trunk weighing down on the head of the femur could be observed when porters were carrying heavy loads of books.[18] The reader's own body could be instructive too – spreading one hand over the cartilages of the false ribs and the other hand at the back of the ribs, and then taking a deep breath, helped with understanding how the ends of the cartilages moved.[19] Pressing on 'the fourth nerve into the arm' (*nervus radialis*) near the elbow (provided there was not too much fat or layers of clothing) would indicate its course, as parts of the finger would go numb.[20] The position of feet in ballet marked *ff* or 'twice simple' showed how far forward the head of the femur could move out of its socket.[21] On one occasion Vesalius referred to himself: at the time of writing the text (he was 26), his 32nd (wisdom) tooth was emerging and it was painful.[22] Individual bodies could thus confirm that knowledge presented in the book was applicable to them.

There were other reasons for introducing individual anecdotes. In describing the size of the lower orifice of the stomach, Vesalius related the story of a 'cunning Spaniard' whom he had encountered recently. In a fit of jealousy, this man had swallowed whole a courtesan's jewellery – a necklace with forty pearls and a gold cross fitted with five gems given to her from another admirer – in the full knowledge that he could pass them through his bowel.[23] Galen had remarked how coins, gold rings and other indigestible objects could be passed through the bowel, but Vesalius's story of the Spanish thief made the point more vividly and consequently more memorably. Vesalius often sought to better Galen's descriptions.

The bodies encountered in the theatre became the basis for a more generalized body in the book. This was an important step in establishing anatomical knowledge that applied to all human bodies. The classical idea of canon helped Vesalius express the idea of a generalized body whose features were determined by observations from dissecting individuals coupled with consideration of function. He also utilized bodies of others he had encountered: thieves, Turks, his distinguished friends, people going about their own business, his readers and even himself. They illustrated acceptable variations, confirmed insights made from cadavers in living bodies and updated classical examples. Both canonical and individual bodies helped to establish a general knowledge of how the body was made.

MALE AND FEMALE BODIES

The additional woodcuts made for *Epitome*, the abridged version of *Fabrica*, are a useful introduction to Vesalius's view on male and female bodies. The male and female nudes (illus. 53) shown in near symmetrical gesture indicate that both male and female bodies needed to be described, rather than letting the male body stand in for both. The gesture of the nude female figure is echoed in the additional sheets of the organs of the male (illus. 56) and the female (illus. 57), though the limbs on the left side were truncated to make space for the additional images.[24] The torso in both sheets consisted of the veins, arteries, lungs and heart. To the left of the full-length figure, both sheets show other structures common to both bodies: the omentum, stomach, liver, and the portal, azygos and intestinal veins. At the top right are the organs of generation – the testes with seminal vessels and the penis with the bladder for the male (illus. 56), and the uterus with the female 'testes' (ovaries to us), 'seminal' vessels and bladder (illus. 57) for the female figure. Vesalius remarked that the names of the

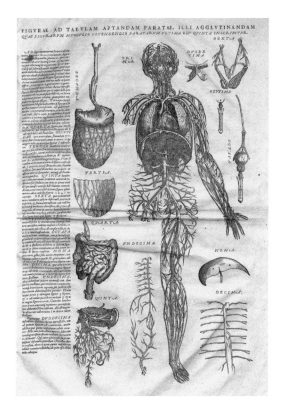

female organs could be otherwise, but because they 'correspond in form and substance' to the male organs, he had adopted the names of the male organs. This was a common view in this period.[25]

Once these sheets were reinforced with sturdier paper from the back, the smaller woodcuts of organs and veins were to be cut out and glued onto the central figure (illus. 4). The male set was then to be attached to the skeleton at the front of the book (illus. 58), and the female layers to the figure of nerves at the end of the book (illus. 59). By this arrangement, Vesalius did not mean that men had bones but no nerves, and women had nerves but no bones. Nobody doubted that both men and women had bones

56 'Shapes prepared to fit the figure which should be glued to the one marked the last or the fifth of the figures showing the muscles [illus. 58].' *Epitome* (1543).

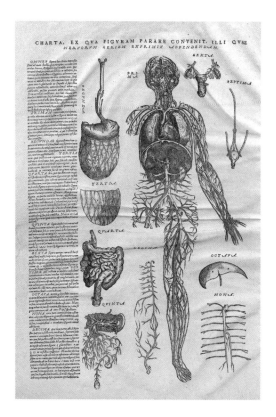

as well as nerves. It was more a way to economize on the number of images (an important point of consideration in *Epitome*), and yet ensure a place for a paper manikin each for a male and a female. These emphasize the point, commonly made in this period and repeated by Vesalius, that God had created man *and* woman and endowed them with different organs of generation for the sake of propagating humankind.[26]

Vesalius's discussion of the organs of generation in *Fabrica* is quite different in tone from the confident, bombastic style of the other parts of the book because he had not been able to dissect enough female cadavers, especially pregnant ones. He described

57 'A sheet from which it is fitting to make a figure which should be attached to the one that shows the course of nerves [illus. 59].' *Epitome* (1543).

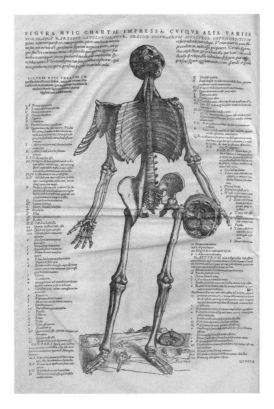

himself as 'storm-tossed on a mighty sea of opinions', reciting from Galen's *On Seeds* the divergence of views with respect to whether both males and females emit semen; the material, derivation and function of semen; the course of seminal vessels; and whether the testes produce semen (as Galen argued) or were a structure to hold down the seminal vessels like a weight that 'weavers attach to their looms' (as the Aristotelians claimed).[27]

Acknowledging that he would not be able to resolve all these points of contention, Vesalius hoped that some clarity could be achieved by describing the anatomical details of the organs, which could be confirmed by dissection. He nevertheless conceded that

58 'The figure printed on this sheet – to which is glued another figure comprised of different parts of the body [illus. 56] – can be counted as the fifth of the figures showing the muscles . . .' *Epitome* (1543).

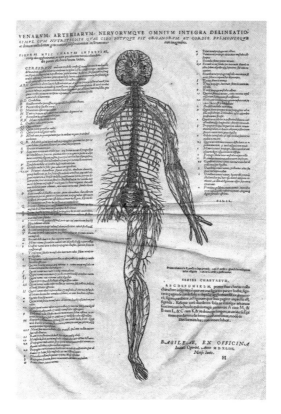

'however carefully you study Nature's handiwork, you will not be able to find a solution that seems sound from every point of view.' He contrasted his humility to the dogmatic clarity claimed by those clinging to the words of another authority.[28] The possibility that nature's 'handiwork' may not reveal everything was not simply a rhetorical ploy but based on his limited access to female cadavers. Unlike Berengario, he had not been able to dissect pregnant or menstruating women.[29]

Vesalius also had difficulty entering the women's world of childbirth. 'Only after much pleading' was he admitted to the homes of Italian women.[30] Vesalius reported with disdain how

59 'A complete delineation of all the veins, arteries and nerves and of the organs of nutrition for food and drink, together with the images of the heart, the lungs and the female organs serving generation [illus. 57].' *Epitome* (1543).

midwives attending such homes made predictions about the future of a baby – for example, the umbilical cord wrapped around the neck meant death by hanging. He was, however, more forgiving of a popular custom of keeping 'the third wrapping of the foetus [amniotic sac]', called in the Low Countries a helmet for boys and a headband for girls. Probably because his mother had kept one, he considered this custom a mark of parental affection rather than superstitious practice: 'I personally think it more elegant if

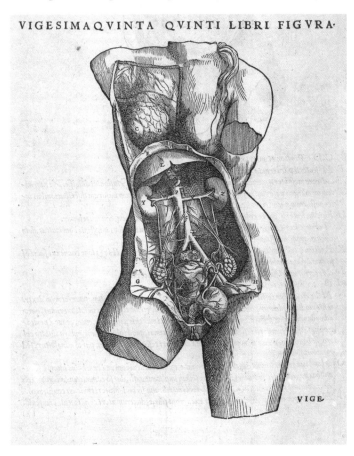

60 'We have reflected the bladder downward to the left side . . . to prevent the bladder from blocking inspecting the uterus.'

these wrappings are given by the mother to the child when they grow up' rather than being tossed out at birth.[31]

Two figures from Book Five (illus. 48 and 60) in *Fabrica* illustrate what was common and different in the male and female viscera.[32] In both figures, remnants of the peritoneum that have been cut away are visible around the edges of the cavity; the liver at the top left of the cavity is shown with the portal vein cut off at the top; the vena cava runs down the trunk with the great artery shown to its right; the blood vessels serving the right kidney (to the left of the image) are placed higher on the vena cava than those serving the left kidney down along the vena cava (the higher right kidney indicates animal anatomy); and the pelvic bones are removed to show a portion of the rectum cut off from the intestines and the ureters running from the kidney to the bladder. In addition, the figure of the female body (illus. 60) shows the ovaries, the uterus and the breast with its glandules. This is also the only instance where, next to the breast, the 'fleshy substance' (*fascia*) – common to both men and women – was shown in *Fabrica*.[33] The male figure (illus. 48) shows parts of the diaphragm and the (broken) ribs, the fatty wrapping of kidneys, the prostate and the testes. A 'soft flaccid penis' was marked 'S', probably deliberately, as Vesalius described it as forming with the bladder the shape of the letter S. The long and winding course of the seminal veins, Vesalius explained, made the blood more refined, and on reaching the testes the seminal arteries and veins spread into thin branches like a net, where the blood was turned into semen.[34]

Given the closeness in structure of the female 'seminal' veins and the male ones, Vesalius sided with Galen (against Aristotle) in the belief that women also produced semen.[35] Drawing a parallel with the liver that produced blood from food that had been refined through long, convoluted intestinal tracts, he wrote:

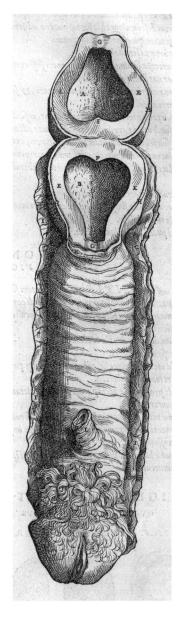

As has been said about the flesh of the liver, so too the substance of the testicle, by a faculty native to itself, bestows the completed nature of semen upon the blood and spirit contained in its small vessels. This force is the cause of ruggedness and virility in men and of womanliness in women; it so alters the entire body that what is by itself neither man nor woman becomes man or woman.[36]

The idea of a sex-neutral physical body that became male or female due to its 'innate faculty' reflects Galen's view that the difference between male and female bodies was a matter of degrees in quality: women were temperamentally 'moister and colder' than men, who were 'drier and hotter'. This accounted for why only half of seminal veins and arteries of men were present in women's 'testes' and why younger or older men might develop breasts since they were 'moister'.[37]

Because of his difficulty accessing pregnant female bodies, modern commentators are agreed that Vesalius's discussion of the female reproductive organs is the least satisfactory section in *Fabrica*.[38] One of the few observations Vesalius did make of the uterus was from a woman who claimed in vain that she was pregnant in the hope of delaying her execution. This was the fact that a uterus

61 'The present figure represents the uterus cut away from the body. It is the same size as we found to be the uterus of a woman quite recently dissected at Padua.'

could stretch 'to an astonishing length', much more so than the male penis.[39] The accompanying image (illus. 61) showed at the top the cross section of a non-pregnant uterus to indicate its shape and the thickness of its tunics, and the actual extent to which its 'neck' (vagina) could stretch out.[40] If not to shock, this life-size image was meant to impress. It certainly caught the attention of several contemporary as well as modern readers.[41]

Beyond the organs of generation, Vesalius noted in *Fabrica* that the shape of pelvic bones was different between men and women, but that the number of teeth was the same.[42] He accepted from Realdo Colombo, 'my good friend' and then professor in the arts faculty at Padua, that the hyoid bone was sometimes covered with a (stylohyoid) ligament in women. His observation that the sagittal suture rarely extended in men and even less often in women led him to declare (against Aristotle) that the skulls of women and men were not permanently different. The male body was not always the default for describing the working of the human body either. For example, periodic haemorrhoids in men were likened to women's menstruation, described as a beneficial form of evacuating excess blood in the body.[43] Vesalius's views cannot easily be reduced to a 'one-sex' model (as some scholars have contended, especially on the basis of similiarity of illus. 61 to the shape of the penis) that took the male body as the norm. As with earlier and contemporary authors, Vesalius tried to understand what was common *and* different between male and female bodies.

GALEN'S BODY – ANIMAL OR HUMAN?

Vesalius sought to establish the canonical human body by frequent dissection and determining the function of parts of the body. What he found, however, was that the human body was not as Galen had described it. For example, the human heart does not have a bone; the sternum is composed of six, not seven segments; the pericardium is attached to the diaphragm; the nerves are not hollow; and haemorrhoid veins are offshoots of the vein between the liver and the spleen, not a branch of the vena cava.[44] Vesalius was proud that he was the first to assign to the ligament in the sole of the foot (*aponeurosis plantaris*) the same role as that of the broad tendon in the hand (*aponeurosis palmaris*).[45] On his own count, Vesalius had corrected Galen in more than two hundred places.

Yet, Vesalius knew that describing a human body that was different from Galen's on the basis of his own observation alone was problematic. Vesalius could be accused of either not looking carefully enough or not knowing his Galen well enough, as Corti had needled him. It was possible – as Vesalius himself suggested – to argue that the human bodies in Galen's time were different from those in his time.[46] To defend his position, Vesalius introduced bodies of animals. Placing the human upper jaw on top of

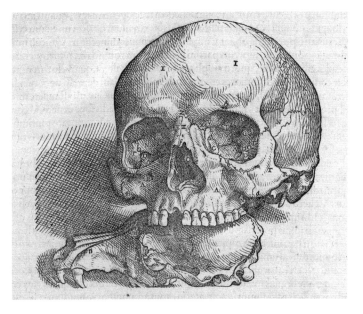

62 'We have portrayed a dog's skull beneath the human one so that Galen's description of bones of the upper jaw may the more easily be understood by anyone.'

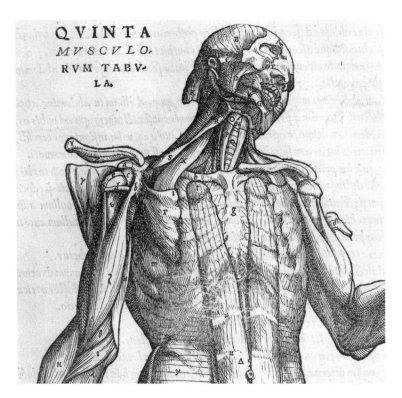

a canine one (illus. 62) enabled Vesalius to make a direct point of comparison.[47] It showed that neither a suture that according to Galen divided the fourth maxillary bone into two ('n' on the canine jaw) nor an extension ('lm' in the canine jaw) of the suture dividing the first and fourth maxillary bones under the eye ('kl' in the canine) was present in the human skull.

Another striking if less obvious illustration was placing a muscle from an animal onto the human body. For example, Galen's 'fifth muscle moving the thorax' matched a simian, not a human one (illus. 63).[48] Rather than just asserting that Galen was simply wrong, Vesalius showed that Galen had dissected an animal – not a human – body. Given that Galen himself had discussed dissecting

63 'r. This delimits the fleshy part of the rectus abdominis . . . In the interval between r and f . . . a tendon, membrane or unfleshed portion of the muscle is noted here belonging to the rectus abdominis of the monkey.'

animals throughout *On Anatomical Procedures* and urged his readers to take the opportunity if they had one to dissect a human body, this was not a difficult point to infer.[49] While animals had been used as proxies in his time when human cadavers for public anatomies were limited, Vesalius now used them in *Fabrica* in another way – as evidence to support his own views. Nobody before Vesalius had taken the meticulous care that he did in checking Galen's description against animal anatomy. He also urged students to dissect humans as well as apes, dogs, birds, fish and reptiles.[50] Many kinds of bodies were mobilized in *Fabrica* in order to establish knowledge about the human body.

Vesalius himself was not free from errors. While in several cases he deliberately introduced animal structures to illustrate the point that the source of Galen's errors was the dissection of animals rather than humans, there was also unacknowledged reliance on animals in *Fabrica*. For example, the images of the hyoid bone and the annular placenta are based on canine anatomy, and those of the arteries are simian.[51] He rejected Galen's 'muscle hidden in the back of the knee' (*musculus popliteus*) as flexing the knee because it was too slight to lift the lower leg and its obliquity could not allow it to move the leg vertically, but Vesalius was also mistaken in claiming that it was not attached to the femur. In various parts of *Fabrica* he followed Galen's descriptions and explanations. Though Vesalius could not find the pores between the ventricles of the heart through which venous blood was believed to seep from the right to the left ventricle, he did not dismantle the whole edifice of Galenic physiology or humoral theory.[52] In other words, he did not come up with a thoroughly modern view of the human body, but it would be harsh to expect one person to accomplish such a feat in a matter of a few years.

Living in the times that he did, Vesalius knew that going against ancient authorities was risky. He introduced the anatomical points that diverged from the views of the revered authorities, and especially Galen, as 'paradoxes'.[53] 'Paradox' was another classical term meaning a contradiction that went against commonly held positions. It should be deemed at least as plausible as accepted opinions. This was a classical expression that put Vesalius's views on a par with those of Galen. But which of them was right could not be established by resorting to another authority. A different kind of adjudicator was needed. When Vesalius noted that the wrapping of the heart (*pericardium*) was attached to the transverse septum (diaphragm) in humans, contrary to what Galen had said, he wrote: 'These facts, which are completely at odds with Galen's opinions and are surprising truths [*paradoxa*] learned from the book of man that tells no lies, must not be passed over.'[54] It is striking that the body here was likened to a book – the emblem of learned medicine. Learned physicians had made themselves learned by reading books. Vesalius's point was that they should also approach the body as if it were a book and learn from it. While a book written by a human author could contain errors, this book of the body, Vesalius claimed, 'told no lies'.

But what about the person who wrote a book based on this 'book of man'? How could the reader of *Fabrica* trust that its author was not mendacious or error-ridden? How did Vesalius present himself to tip the balance of paradoxes in his favour?

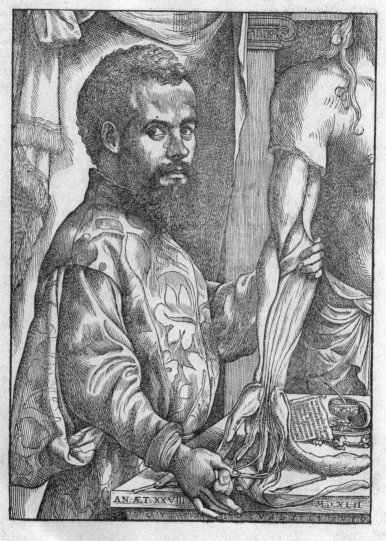

AN·ÆT·XXVIII   M·D·XLII

EIGHT

Vesalius: Surgeon, Anatomist, Physician?

esalius relocated his arena of debate from the theatre to the book in order to establish his view of the human body against Galen's. He had to find a way of tipping the readers' opinion in his favour. What authority did he have to make such claims? Vesalius described himself on the title page of *Fabrica* as 'professor at the school of physicians at Padua' (illus. 1). The job title was correct, but we also know that his professorship was in surgery, the least well-paid post in the medical faculty and much less prestigious than the other professors in medicine. He had to present himself carefully to the reader – as a surgeon, or an anatomist, or a physician? None of these seemed suitable.

SURGEON?

In the preface addressed to the emperor, Vesalius briefly described his career to date: as a student at Paris, he attended public dissections performed so carelessly by barbers that he was forced to take the matter into his own hands. He learned how to dissect and was already dissecting at the third demonstration he had ever attended.[1] He then honed his dissecting skills at Louvain, where anatomical knowledge came to be acknowledged as a foundation for philosophy, thanks to him. And now at Padua, 'the world's most famous university', Vesalius described himself as continuing

64 Vesalius at the age of 28 in 1542.

his 'inquiry into the construction of the human frame', because anatomy was pertinent also to 'the profession of surgical medicine' (*professionem chirurgicae medicinae*), which (as he continued in brackets) he had been teaching for five years, having been granted a stipend from the 'illustrious Venetian Senate'. With a tinge of defensiveness, he added that he had been lecturing on surgery so as 'not to divorce myself completely from the rest of medicine'. Clearly, Vesalius did not want his readers to think that lecturing on surgery at Padua was the desired end point or pinnacle of his career.

The Latin term for surgeon, *chirurgus*, is a transliteration of the Greek word meaning someone who worked with their hands. According to Vesalius, surgeons were that group of practitioners whom university-educated physicians looked down upon as less respectable than even their own servants, and to whom they had relegated the manual work. It was not, however, the socially inferior profession of the surgeon that Vesalius was trying to elevate. He did not disparage surgeons openly but did not expect them to be familiar with humanist scholarship either – as he noted, surgeons in his own day used the Arabic term 'zirbus' for the omentum.[2]

In *Fabrica*, surgeons or surgical procedures were mentioned only sporadically. When Vesalius did refer to surgical procedures, it was to ram home the importance of anatomical knowledge. Familiarity with the sutures of the skull was necessary when applying cautery (a piece of heated iron); the course of nerves had to be understood accurately to avoid damaging them when applying caustic remedies; veins supported by fleshy membranes had to be cut when bloodletting sick patients; and the direction of muscles fibres had to be taken into consideration when removing abscesses of glands so as to prevent wrinkling of the skin in the neck. There were many useful points of this kind that he could offer, but they were not the main focus of *Fabrica*. In fact, he thought it 'ridiculous to mix up other branches of medicine with this anatomical branch'.[3] Anatomical knowledge was certainly necessary for surgeons, but *Fabrica* was not a textbook about surgery.

This may explain why surgical procedures were not shown in the main illustrations of *Fabrica*, though they formed the background scene to some of the decorative initials. The initial H (illus. 65), for example, shows cauterization.[4] A seated patient is held steady by a man from behind; the surgeon holds in his right hand a cautery and in his left hand a plate with holes through which the tip of the cautery was applied; a putto to the right is tending a fire to heat the cautery.

The index of *Fabrica* listed only one entry under surgery (*chirurgia*): the 'delineation of instruments of surgery'. This referred to the initials E and F printed together without forming a word in order to show the instrument for correcting dislocated bones (illus. 31).[5] The relegation of the depiction of surgical procedures

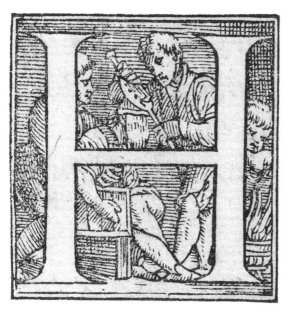

65 'This is the point to which doctors apply what is popularly known as a cautery, consisting of a piece of candescent gold or iron ... this involves considerable risk.' Woodcut 3.7 centimetres/1½ in. square.

to the initials reflected Vesalius's priorities. Stitching up intestines or abdominal wounds could be practised on live animals, but Vesalius saw such an exercise as more appropriate for training the hand rather than investigating the function of organs.[6] Function, as noted in the previous chapter, was essential in determining the shape and structure of the human body. It was what made anatomy a philosophical discipline. Vesalius wanted to align anatomy with a discipline with a higher status, natural philosophy, away from the lower status of the craft of surgery. This implied that a surgeon's manual skill was not sufficient for acquiring sound anatomical knowledge.

ANATOMIST?

Distancing himself from surgery did not mean, however, that Vesalius could do without instruments. He included a woodcut of what he called 'anatomical' instruments (illus. 66).[7] These were readily available tools used by other craftsmen or from everyday life rather than bespoke instruments. Shown on the table were barbers' razors for shaving, saws used by comb-makers, small knives for cutting reed pens, common table knives, bookbinding cords (those from Germany were the best, Vesalius said), hooks made from table forks, and curved needles made by bending ordinary, straight ones. These had various uses. Intestines should be sewn up with a large needle bent into a curve and bookbinding thread; small pen-cutting knives were useful for dissecting the muscles of the eyelid and other delicate structures; a hollow reed pipe was used to inflate intestines or lungs; a hammer and a stout knife were needed when dividing the lower jaw bones.[8] Existing implements made and used for other purposes could thus become 'anatomical' instruments. These were a far cry from Berengario's bespoke instruments that might be used only once to treat a specific injury (illus. 15).

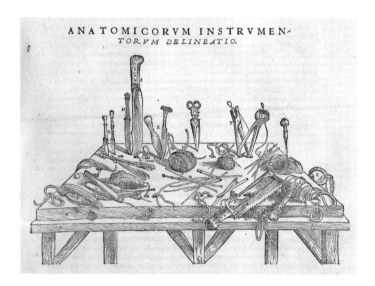

ANATOMICORVM INSTRVMEN-
TORVM DELINEATIO.

Not all of the instruments on the table were actually used by Vesalius in his public dissections.[9] Nor was he wedded to using particular instruments for specific procedures since the hand could do some of the work equally well. A fingertip could be used for lifting skin or for separating membranes instead of a hook, a small boxwood knife or a razor, and the whole hand was just as effective as a blunt knife in separating muscles.[10]

While Vesalius gave the impression that dissection was less dependent on specific instruments, he was also clear that some skill was required to use them effectively. Unfortunately, as Vesalius lamented, dissecting skill among medical students was poor to non-existent at the time. They would do well, he remarked, to learn from butchers how to flay skin, scorch cuticles or remove cartilages or larynxes.[11] But a butcher's method was also rather crude and did not require much finesse.[12] There were levels of difficulty: dissecting the nerves and vessels was harder than dissecting muscles. 'The most troublesome and difficult incision in the whole body' was separating from the concave part of the liver

66 'Delineation of anatomical instruments'. Compare illus. 31 showing a *surgical* instrument.

the branches of (hepatic) nerves overlying arterial branches (*arteria hepatica propria*), under which was the gall bladder duct (*ductus cysticus*) that further needed to be separated from the portal vein.[13]

But the ability to dissect did not in itself guarantee correct knowledge. Inattentive dissectors could miss the correct place of insertion of a muscle; careful dissectors could still mistake fat for part of the urinary channel; and even experienced dissectors could err if they were dissecting only the body of an animal.[14] This may be why the actual procedures of dissection using these instruments were not shown in the main illustrations. Instead, it is in the background of the initial D that a putto is shown holding a severed head while another places a saw along a horizontal line marked across it (illus. 67). This closely resembled Vesalius's instruction about marking a line across the forehead with a carpenter's cord soaked in dye.[15] He also noted that a sickle-like saw that mimicked the shape of the brain was of no use – perhaps an oblique reference to Dryander's 'orbicular saw' (illus. 19).[16] *Fabrica*'s main illustrations instead showed the *result* of the dissections using these anatomical

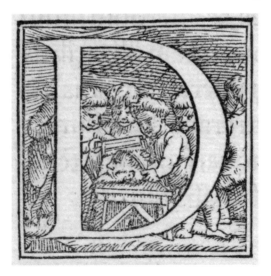

67 Do not remove the hair of the head, 'so you may hold the head more easily with your other hand and both of your partner's hands to keep the head from moving under the saw'. Woodcut 3.7 centimetres/1½ in. square.

instruments. The actual process of dissection was relegated to the initials with a group of putti.

The instruments on the table were 'anatomical' not because they were bespoke tools for specific procedures. What made them 'anatomical' was that they enabled competent dissection that resulted in reliable anatomical knowledge. This anatomical knowledge did not always lead to applications in surgery or treatment. Vesalius pointed out that dissection could reveal knowledge that was not immediately useful (*inutile*).[17] This may be a clue as to why Vesalius was vague about whom he considered to be 'anatomists' (*anatomici*).

In the index to *Fabrica*, six instances of 'anatomists' were listed for their errors, who turn out to be unnamed people described as 'writers', 'followers of Galen' or 'professors of dissections'.[18] Vesalius interchangeably used 'professors of dissection' and 'professors of anatomy' to refer to those who had dissected and expressed views (not always correctly) about the form or function of parts of the human body. His evaluation of them followed a roughly chronological order. Under 'ancient professors of dissection', Vesalius grouped writers spanning five centuries from Herophilus (third century BCE) to Marinus (second century CE). Though their works were mainly known through Galen's criticism of them, they were authorities more ancient than Galen and served as a foil against him.[19] Galen himself was described as foremost among the professors of dissection as well as of anatomists, notwithstanding his mistakes.[20] Then there were others who lived later than Galen who blindly followed Galen and others.[21] This fits into the general chronology presented in the preface to *Fabrica* that anatomical knowledge had declined over time since the ancient Greeks. Vesalius never explicitly identified himself as an anatomist or a professor of dissection in *Fabrica*, however.

PHYSICIAN?

If 'anatomists' did not always get it right, physicians (*medici*) were even worse. They were not just ignorant of dissection.[22] They were pretenders to knowledge, capable of nothing yet quick to disparage the work of others; they were 'windbags' who deemed the only worthy contribution to medicine to be theoretical (whether medicine was an art or a science, for example); they were 'goatish physicians' who hated him so much that they would not miss a chance to make false accusations if they could slander him; they were 'scolds' who heaped wrath on him with 'weird histrionics' if they could justify Galen's errors 'with silly rationalizations'; and they expected to publish with impunity while objecting to Vesalius publishing his views. In short, the learned physicians were guilty of double standards, hypocrisy, jealousy and silliness, in addition to being unable to dissect. Their ultimate fault was their unquestioning allegiance to Galen – a kind of devotion (the Latin word Vesalius used for devotion was *religio*). As his harsh words indicate, Vesalius had strong views against them.

There were two reasons for this. The first was his encounter with Matteo Corti, acknowledged as the greatest Galenist of his time. We recall that Vesalius and Corti disagreed about the authority of Galen in the anatomy theatre at Bologna. As noted by the historian Andrew Cunningham, the two were completely at cross purposes: they did not agree on the basic rules of engagement.[23] In his arena – the theatre – Vesalius could not win over Corti because Corti did not consider himself an anatomist. This may be another reason for Vesalius's ambivalence towards the label of *anatomici*. Heseler described those tasked to conduct the cutting of the body at Bologna as the 'anatomy masters' (*domini anatomistae*).[24] He called Vesalius 'Corti's anatomist' and Corti introduced Vesalius – with a hint of condescension – as 'our dissector' (*noster sector*).[25] At this time an anatomist (*anatomicus*) was too closely linked to the manual aspect of dissection and remained inferior in status to the professor of medicine.

Another reason was more personal. Vesalius used to be one of those ardent followers of Galen who believed in the existence of the *rete mirabile* in the human head. He had even shown the structure in his *Anatomical Tables* (B in illus. 25). Vesalius appears not to have known that Berengario had already denied its existence, or at least did not believe it to be the case until a moment of his own revelation. We do not know exactly when this was, but it must have been soon after his visit to Bologna, since Heseler recorded that Vesalius showed the *rete mirabile* using the head of a sheep without commenting that it did not exist in humans.[26]

Vesalius was thus one of those very people who covered up the fact that he could not see in the human body what Galen had described, as he confessed:

> I myself cannot be sufficiently astonished at my own stupidity and excessive faith in the writings of Galen and other Anatomists, I *who have labored so hard in my devotion to Galen that I never undertook to demonstrate the human head in public dissections without having the head of a lamb or a cow available so I could pluck from the ovine head what I did not find in the human, fool the spectators, and avoid having it said that I did not find the network best known by name to all.*[27]

As this discovery was relatively recent, he urged students who had not attended his public anatomies in the previous two years to attend another and examine it with their own eyes – an act he expressed with the Greek word *autopsia*.[28] This is a rare occasion when Vesalius used this Greek term meaning 'seeing for oneself'. It may appear odd that this phrase was not used more often by Vesalius, but at the time it was a word associated negatively with the empirical sect that Galen criticized for ignoring causal investigation.[29] On this occasion, however, the use of the word *autopsy* was justified as Vesalius was urging students to look at the body, compare Galen's description with his, and judge for themselves whether an anatomical structure existed at all. Perhaps the depiction of the spectator with a magnifying glass (illus. 5) was a veiled criticism of Massa, who recommended the use of spectacles to look for the *rete mirabile*. No manner of magnifying glass would have helped because the *rete mirabile* did not exist in humans.

One of Corti's criticisms that must have rankled with Vesalius was that his knowledge of Galen was deficient. A demonstration of his humanist credentials was therefore in order. In *Fabrica*, he let it be known that he had been part of da Monte's project of translating Galen's works into Latin from the Greek, had consulted manuscripts and was able to correct mistranslations and misunderstandings: for example, 'hyoid' meant resembling the Greek letter upsilon (υ), not a pig ('hys' in Greek); the confusion of 'glottis' with 'epiglottis' could be traced to transcription errors by the scribes of Galen's Greek manuscripts, compounded by a further misunderstanding by Celsus, repeated in Theodore Gaza's recent translation of Aristotle; Galen's own inconsistent terminology had also added some confusion – the same part of the scapula (*processus coracoideus*) was described as a sigmoid (resembling an old form of the Greek capital of sigma that looks like a roman majuscule C), ankyroid (like the prongs of the anchor which buries itself in the sand) or coracoid (like a crow's beak).[30]

Vesalius also knew that not all works of Galen had survived. Given that Avicenna was familiar with the parts now missing from Galen's *On Anatomical Procedures*, and other lost works of Galen on muscles, Vesalius wondered if those manuscripts might still be found in Bukhara where Avicenna lived.[31] It was also possible, Vesalius posited, that Avicenna knew about Galen's views via another author, such as Oribasius (c. 320–403), who had compiled excerpts from earlier medical authors. Vesalius could furthermore tell that Galen's knowledge and dissecting skills had improved over time, which accounted for some differences between *On the Usefulness of the Parts* and *On Anatomical Procedures*. He suspected that Galen had made some annotations in his own copy of *On the Usefulness of the Parts* but had never revised it thoroughly. These points served to highlight that Vesalius had a good grasp of the Galenic corpus and its transmission, and that he could judge appropriately the different types and sources of confusion in the Galenic text. In other words, Vesalius wanted to show that he knew his Galen well.

THEOLOGIANS

Vesalius also had something to say about theologians. We have already seen him exclude the bodies of Christ and Adam from his discussion. In the case of the two hard sesamoid bones in the toe that looked like hulled chickpeas, Vesalius mentioned the popular belief that they were considered indestructible and could therefore be used to resurrect the body.[32] Belief in the power of these bones as 'seeds of resurrection' was such that three women in Venice had recently ripped the heart out of a boy while he was still alive so as to join it with this ossicle. The women were executed for their crime. Vesalius stated he would not offer his opinion on the alleged marvellous powers of these bones because theologians claimed the sole authority to pronounce on matters of resurrection and immortality. Yet he swiftly added that he had seen these bones many times himself and that they could be broken and burned just like any other bone. Belief in the special powers of these ossicles was based on the idea that they were indestructible, which could readily be refuted on physical grounds. Vesalius was perfectly qualified to make this point.

Vesalius's incidental references to the mistress of a monk (who was expected to lead a life of celibacy) and theologians' special interest in the organs of generation further suggest that he did not believe in blind deference to theologians' authority, even in relation to topics related to the function of the soul. The soul, in the classical sense of the word, was a principle of life, which in turn maintained various physical functions such as nutrition, respiration and sensation exercised by means of physical organs such as the stomach, lungs and nerves. Vesalius objected to the fact that any discussion about the function of the soul might attract accusations from 'censors of our most holy and true religion' of impiety or doubting resurrection.[33] In physical terms, it was right and proper that the physician (*medicus*) should examine the organs and function of the soul. For example, the anatomical structure of the heart indicated that it was the source of the 'vital function' (illus. 25) of distributing the 'vivifying spirit' in the blood to the whole of the body and fomenting innate heat.[34]

As Vesalius had complained about theologians teaching with Reisch's textbook (illus. 20), they knew next to nothing about the physical structure of the human brain, and yet felt entitled to assign various functions of the soul to its parts. Though it had long been assumed by theologians and philosophers that the ventricles of the brain were the physical location of activities such as imagination, reckoning and memory, Vesalius conceded that he could not explain how the brain performed those functions. Reason, considered unique to humans, was often equated with the immortal Christian soul. Anatomically speaking, however, this special status of the human rational soul could not be demonstrated in the brain, because, apart from their size, Vesalius detected virtually no difference between the brains of humans and of animals.[35] Here, Vesalius was careful to draw a line – that the immortality of the human soul remained a mystery, and that the best he could do was to give thanks to the almighty Creator and study as well as possible the design of the physical body.[36] While Vesalius was willing to push at the boundaries between theologians and physicians and stake his claim of competence where possible, he also acknowledged that there were some matters beyond his ken.

TRUTH

The sparse mention of surgeons in *Fabrica* was deliberate, given their lower status in academic medicine. Anatomists could get things wrong if they were inattentive or careless, or did not dissect human bodies or followed Galen glibly. With a tinge of the zeal of a former believer-turned-unbeliever, Vesalius lambasted the physicians as even worse, because they believed Galen without dissection. And theologians had no business claiming expertise over the physical body. No single authority or profession sufficed as a model with whom Vesalius could identify. All were prone to errors in establishing reliable knowledge of the human body.

While Vesalius found no satisfactory model to follow among his contemporaries, it is possible to make a case – ironically – that Vesalius fashioned himself after Galen, as argued by Cunningham.[37] In noting Galen's lengthy refutation of a misunderstanding by Aristotle, Vesalius suggested that Aristotle's followers should turn the table on Galen by personally dissecting the human body and charging Galen with what Galen had charged others with.[38] Vesalius himself practised this, by challenging his students to dissect bodies themselves in order to 'discover whether I was wrong'.[39] Galen had lambasted those pontificating aloft in a chair without doing any dissection and pointed out the errors of his predecessors based on his own experience. Vesalius too made these points. He even declared that Galen's 'ghost' would, if not approve, at least not be angry with him for revealing that Galen had used the body of an ape, because they both strove to improve anatomical knowledge.[40]

Vesalius contrasted his approach of examining directly the human body with swearing 'by somebody's words more than you should'.[41] This phrase evoked the well-known declaration by the Roman poet Horace (65–8 BCE) when he abandoned poetry in favour of philosophy that he would not be 'bound over to swear as any Master dictates'.[42] The shortened version of the Latin, 'nullius in verba', became the motto of the Royal Society of London, founded in 1660.[43] We tend to think of anti-authoritarian attitudes as modern, but this too was a well-known classical trope.[44]

Ultimately, Vesalius posited a value beyond human authority – truth. Those who could appreciate Vesalius's attempt to rise above professional jealousies and rivalries were those drawn to the love of truth.[45] It is for them, he declared, that the book was written and he cared for their endorsement alone. This was an elaboration of what Massa and Berengario had already expressed, namely the value of 'truth' over authorities. True knowledge of the human body could not be attained by cleaving to the words of others. There had to be a different way. What was involved in such a way can be gleaned from his portrait.

THE PORTRAIT

Vesalius's portrait (illus. 64) is another carefully staged composition which should not be taken as representing an actual scene. It was designed to convey certain points about the person portrayed, and it is a clue to his identity and his values. He is shown standing in front of a draped curtain, behind which is a column with a scroll-patterned head that makes it an Ionic column. These were common background props for portraiture in this period, and used also by Jan Steven van Calcar, who probably designed this portrait.[46] Vesalius is shown holding a dissected arm of an upright body, only part of whose torso is shown. On the table, there is a quill in an elaborate inkpot on a stand; next to it is a piece of paper with writing; a knife is placed towards the edge of the table; and a razor with a handle is visible under Vesalius's right hand.

On the edge of the table is written, 'age 28 in 1542' (*An[no] Aet[atis] XXVIII MDXLII*), another common convention in portraiture to indicate the age of the person portrayed.

Vesalius's gesture corresponds to his own instructions about dissecting the 'first muscle moving the fingers' (*musculus flexor digitorum superficialis*).[47] Detach the head of the muscle, pull it towards oneself, and lift it from the groove of the carpus so as to reveal the tendons stretching to the four fingers, each of which has a perforation through which the tendon of the 'second muscle moving the fingers' (*musculus flexor digitorum profundus*) under the first muscle passes through. The text on the piece of paper on the table is headed 'Of the muscles moving the figures, chapter 30', an earlier version of what became chapter 43 of Book Two describing these muscles.[48] There, Vesalius explained that because the bones of the fingers did not have the breadth to house the tendons of the 'first' and 'second' muscles side by side, the Maker of all things had with 'astounding ingenuity' stacked them on top of each other with perforations that let those below pass through.[49] Vesalius was thus showing off God's ingenious creation through the arm he had dissected.

A striking feature of this portrait is that Vesalius does not hold an instrument – neither the quill nor the knife – in his hand. His hands hold the arm and the muscles, and the instruments rest on the table. This is not the case in the frontispiece (illus. 1), where Vesalius is shown holding a knife in the hand that he rests on the body, though the table similarly displays an inkstand with a quill as well as some cutting tools. The emphasis is on the display of the dissected female body rather than on the act of dissection.[50]

In the close-up portrait (illus. 64), Vesalius cannot be tied solely to the figure of a dissector or an author. In fact, the illustrations in *Fabrica* never show Vesalius 'in action', sleeves rolled up, cutting into a body with an instrument in his hand. We can spot small hints of the process of dissection such as a blood vessel or a colon tied up with cord. But we do not see the dissector's hands, which is probably deliberate. The one picture that Vesalius mentioned that he decided *not* to use would have shown an assistant's hands, though the immediate reason for rejecting the image was that it was too difficult to represent a very thin membrane (*septum pellucidum*).

What happened in the anatomy theatre – such as sawing through a skull (illus. 67) or inflating a lung – was relegated to the initials showing putti in action. The putti perform the manual work involved in first-hand dissection that Vesalius urged medical students to do, but their nakedness also has the effect of shifting attention away from who should be doing the work to the procedure itself.[51] As letters, the initials were part of the words that made up the text that described the form and function of the dissected parts. The background scenes of these initials were a reminder of the manual work that underpinned what was described in the text. The work of the hand in dissecting and writing was thus integrated on the page.

In the portrait, Vesalius is not shown 'at work' with his hands, but it is his handiwork – both the dissected body and his writing – that is displayed.[52] It suggests the equal weight Vesalius attached to the dissection of the body and writing about the body. Dissection was needed to understand how the body was made, and writing was needed to explain why the body was made in the way that it was. His hands touch the dissected arm to guide the viewers' eyes to the source and adjudicator of anatomical knowledge.

Quite literally overshadowed by what is going on above the table, on the side underneath the table and on the edge of the image is an inscription. Scholars have identified it as a modified version of a motto about treating patients attributed by Celsus to the ancient Greek physician Asclepiades.[53] Celsus's version reads 'safely, swiftly, pleasantly' (*tuto, celeriter, juncunde*) and the inscription in the portrait, 'more swiftly, pleasantly and safely' (*ocyus, iucunde et tuto*). It may well express an aspiration to treat patients more quickly than the famed ancient physician, or that anatomical knowledge would lead to swifter healing. Its position in the shadows suggests that this point was secondary to what was going on above: establishing true knowledge of human anatomy.

It was important that this anatomical knowledge was presented in a book, the hallmark of the learned physician. Corti had refused to accept Vesalius's claim in the anatomical theatre because Corti was no anatomist. Vesalius took his argument to the arena of the learned physician. In *Fabrica*, Vesalius described how he dissected the human body, established the functions of parts of the body, and demonstrated the humanist skills required to understand the texts of Galen like any other learned physician. It was not the socially inferior profession of the surgeon that Vesalius was trying to elevate. Vesalius wanted to restore anatomical knowledge to its rightful place among knowledge professed by the learned physicians.

NINE

Making and Unmaking

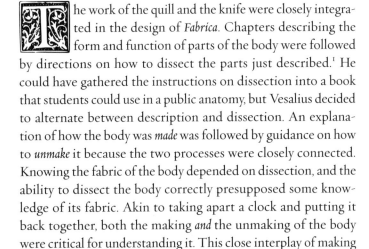he work of the quill and the knife were closely integra-
ted in the design of *Fabrica*. Chapters describing the
form and function of parts of the body were followed
by directions on how to dissect the parts just described.[1] He
could have gathered the instructions on dissection into a book
that students could use in a public anatomy, but Vesalius decided
to alternate between description and dissection. An explanation of how the body was *made* was followed by guidance on how
to *unmake* it because the two processes were closely connected.
Knowing the fabric of the body depended on dissection, and the
ability to dissect the body correctly presupposed some knowledge of its fabric. Akin to taking apart a clock and putting it
back together, both the making *and* the unmaking of the body
were critical for understanding it. This close interplay of making
and unmaking the body was a central feature of both *Fabrica* and
Epitome.

THE MAKING OF THE HUMAN BODY

Each chapter of each book of *Fabrica* began by describing how
parts of the body were made in order to fulfil certain functions.
Such a description was informed by insights from dissection. For
example, the 'fourth muscle moving the arm' (*musculus latissimus
dorsi*) was not attached to the scapula with fibres, and therefore

could not have the function of moving the scapula (a view Vesalius attributed to Galen); the absence of a membranous sieve in the middle of the kidney indicated that the function of filtering blood into urine was located in the fleshy substance of the kidney; and the fact that the hemorrhoidal veins originated not in the vena cava but in the portal vein meant it had the function of discharging black bile that could not be absorbed by the spleen.[2]

Rather than merely assert the shape and function of parts of the human body solely on the basis of what he found in a dissection, however, Vesalius bolstered his explanation using another classical trope – analogy with artefacts. Aristotle had famously illustrated his four causes of nature by reference to house-building: the material cause was like the bricks and wood for the house; the formal cause the design of the house in the mind of the builder; the efficient cause the art of building; and shelter was the final cause or the purpose of the house that was built. Galen likened the bones to the walls of a house, the spine to the keel of a ship, the omentum to a pouch, and the round apertures of the cervical vertebrae (*foramina transversaria*) to polished perforations made by woodcarvers.[3] Such analogies emphasized the idea that objects and processes in nature had been made deliberately and skilfully by nature, often identified with a 'maker'. Vesalius used such tropes extensively, improving or updating classical ones and adding his own examples.

Galen, for instance, had invoked the 'three-grooved' barb of a dart to describe the three 'processes' in the right ventricle of the heart (*valva atrioventricularis dextra*). Vesalius updated this analogy using the tip of an armour-piercing Turkish spear. He added – probably because he thought his readers might not know what a Turkish spearpoint looked like – an explanation of its manufacture: to make the 'long iron point less heavy and the angles sharper, they file down a groove between the two angles so that as the spearhead comes to a point from its base, it shows three angles and the same numbers of grooves'.[4] By updating Galen's description in striking contemporary terms, Vesalius rendered the shape of the tricuspid valves more memorable. In *On the Usefulness of the Parts*, where the three-grooved dart was mentioned, Galen remarked that another opening into the left ventricle of the heart that divided into two processes (*valva atrioventricularis sinistra*) had not been compared to any known object. Vesalius promptly provided one – it looked like a bishop's mitre, and we now know it as the mitral valve.[5]

Vesalius introduced more analogies of his own. The septum (*septum pellucidum*) between the left and the right hemispheres of the brain was translucent like the thin specular stones used by Italian master builders for windows and doors, or like 'a damp host that priests are accustomed to administer at mass'.[6] The small bones in the ear unknown to the ancients and therefore without a name were named after their shapes resembling a hammer (*malleus*) and anvil (*incus*), names still in use today.[7] In choosing the best analogy for the interlocking of the sutures of the skull, Vesalius listed four types of joints: teeth of saws facing each other, fingernail-shaped rims with matching undulation, a chest with dovetailed joints and a decorative hem (illus. 68).[8] For Vesalius, the dovetailed joint more accurately described the sutures than the fingernail-shaped joints, but the best likeness was the florets sewn onto the hems of women's garments. This may have been a silent correction of Berengario, who had described the sutures of the skull as similar to dovetailed joints.

A bishop's mitre, a communion wafer or a floral hem would have been familiar enough for readers to be able to imagine analogous structures, but Turkish artefacts less so. Vesalius wrote that the innominate cartilage of the larynx (*cartilago cricoidea*) looked like a thumb ring used by Turkish archers, and the auricles of the heart resembled the leather bags sewn on each side of a Turkish saddle that inflated when swimming across rivers on

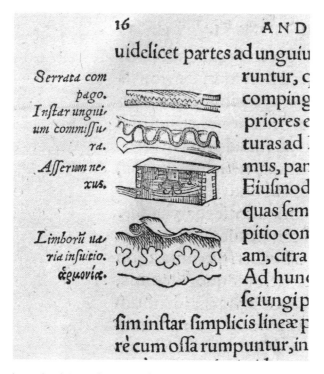

horseback.[9] Analogies with Turkish artefacts had the additional effect of demonstrating Vesalius's familiarity with exotic cultural objects that fascinated European elites at the time. Another, somewhat forced likeness between 'the fleshy outer circle of the diaphragm' (*diaphragma, pars costalis*) and a tennis racket crushed on its sides was also a cue to his readers who knew the emerging sport of tennis that Vesalius too was familiar with that fashionable pastime.[10]

Vesalius also appeared to suggest that human artefacts had been inspired by nature's clever constructions of the human body. Craftsmen had applied the structure of the larynx to wind instruments; the viscid liquid covering a 'ligament [hyaline cartilage] of the tenth muscle of the thigh' (*musculus obturator internus*) had

---

68 'The suture, for which the Greek word is *rhaphe*, is a type of joint which resembles two things sewn together.'

been copied in pulleys so that ropes would last longer; the commingling of the nerves in the upper arm (*plexus brachialis*) was so elegant 'that artisans could first have learned from its appearance' to weave 'the thin cords hung from the hats of Cardinals'.[11] And perhaps somewhat in jest, Vesalius suggested that his readers might think that 'the Franciscans, Jacobites and especially the Benedictines borrowed the shape of their cowl' from 'the second muscle moving the scapula' (*musculus trapezius*) that covered part of the back of the neck and hugged the shoulder.[12] A friar in profile shown in the frontispiece could be referring to this point (illus. 5).[13] It is unlikely that Vesalius thought that those who initially designed instruments, pulleys, cardinals' hats or friars' cowls were actual dissectors, but these were striking rhetorical moves that tightened the parallel between artefacts and the human body.

Manufacturing processes could, furthermore, illuminate some finer points of morphology. For example, the cavities on both sides of the nose (*sinus paranasales*) were likened to what was left hollow during a casting process (after a wax shape inside a plaster cast had been melted away). This 'lost-wax technique' was in regular use by contemporary sculptors, including Agostino Zoppo, who was active in Padua at the time.[14] A humoral part of the eye (*corpus vitreum*) resembled two states of glass in colour and clarity: it was like 'chilled white glass', but in consistency it resembled glass 'that has been liquefied in furnaces, which we see covering the iron pipes on which it is removed from the furnace by artisans', though such molten glass was 'red-hot iron' in colour.[15] Vesalius could have observed glass-making in Murano.

The human body as something that was made implied that it had a maker. Nature thus operated like a craftsman. It was described as fashioning, contriving, creating, carving out and engraving the body with incredible skill, 'no mean cleverness' and foresight; and the human body was nature's 'handiwork'.[16] Just as Galen used the terms 'nature' and 'creator' interchangeably, Vesalius also invoked a creator. It was the Maker who made the eye rotate for wider vision; the Architect who built organs of nutrition; and the supreme Maker of all things who contrived the respiratory organs.[17]

Conversely, this meant that erroneous anatomical structures were a challenge to the competence of nature as a craftsman – for example, attributing to the double joint of the head with the first vertebra (*articulatio atlantooccipitalis*) a sideways movement of the head was tantamount to imputing 'negligence to the infinite Author of things', and Galen's erroneous description of the styloid process meant that nature was encumbered with a 'most uncraftsmanlike' structure.[18] The point that erroneous anatomical structures were an affront to God was not new to Vesalius – Galen too had used the same argument.[19] Vesalius updated and redeployed classical strategies available to him to defend his views of why parts of the human body were made in the way that they were.

THE UNMAKING OF THE HUMAN BODY

In *Fabrica*, dissection was not presented as a process of discovery from scratch by someone who knew nothing about the human body. Some prior knowledge of what was being dissected was necessary. Those 'inexperienced' in dissection could miss the bladder if they did not know that it was attached to the peritoneum; the membrane (*facia superficialis*) under the skin could be removed with the fat if its existence was not known; and the muscles 'moving the scapula' could not be dissected before the muscles moving the humerus.[20] Frequent reminders of the number of muscles about to be dissected, and warnings not to remove adjacent or underlying muscles by mistake, indicate how those dissecting the body needed to have a fair idea of what they were about to dissect.[21] The descriptions preceding the instructions on dissection served this purpose.

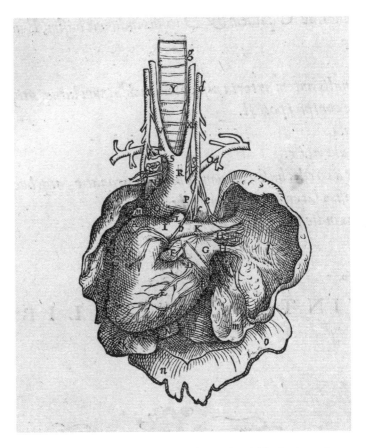

Further guidance on what students should be looking for in the dissected body was provided in the illustrations. Comparing a dissected heart with a corresponding figure (illus. 69) could help them identify the recurrent nerves and arteries (*arteriae carotides communes*).[22] The dissection of the veins, arteries and nerves would be easier if they had consulted the images and explanations from *Epitome*.[23] On another occasion, they were invited to take a skull in their hand, compare it with the woodcut (illus. 62), and then trace the sutures with a quill.[24] Images thus furnished

69 'Take the heart in your hand . . . The great artery (O) is seen in the middle of the base of the heart, partly hidden under the arterial vein (I). When you first see it, compare the dissection with our picture . . .'

students with an understanding of the structure of the body they were dissecting.

Dissection, furthermore, was not a simple sequential dismantling of parts of the body. Vesalius often suggested removing a muscle only from one end and letting it hang over from the other end so that the inner side of the muscle could be examined and its movement checked by pulling on the separated end, before putting the muscle back in place in order to be reminded how the parts were placed together.[25] Dissection was a structured way of learning how the body was made. Parts of the body were tentatively cut out to enable examination of morphological details and functions, and putting them back in situ served as a reminder of their initial position and connections before eventually removing them and proceeding to the next part. To the extent that incisions and separations of parts of the body presupposed a certain amount of knowledge about those parts, and examination of the dissected parts in and out of place confirmed how the parts fitted and functioned together, Vesalius's dissection was a form of *unmaking*.

Too much prior knowledge could be a hindrance in dissection, however, especially if it relied on a single authority. As Vesalius warned, 'if you believe in Galen, you will accuse yourself of carelessness and ignorance in your own dissections.'[26] Instead, Vesalius urged students to determine in their own dissections whether Galen's or his description was correct. For example, students had to decide whether the head of the third muscle moving the lower leg (*musculus semitendinosus*) lay on top of the head of the fourth muscle (*musculus biceps femoris*) (Vesalius's position) or under it (Galen's position).[27] They also needed to know what was said by Galen in order to confirm in their dissection the absence of structures, such as one of the muscles that Galen described as raising the scapula present in an ape but not in humans.[28] Occasionally, Vesalius included a figure of an imaginary structure to indicate what something described by Galen might look like. Comparing such a figure with the dissected body could thus help determine the absence of a particular structure.[29]

For Vesalius dissection was not just about learning how the body was made, but also about determining whose knowledge of the human body was correct. In this process of adjudication, Vesalius enjoined students to dissect with their fellow medical students and decide.[30] This was a social point in that students, not servants, were deemed capable of judging what was correct knowledge. It was also about collective study. Just as the pictorial initials showing dissection scenes have putti in groups, so also were students expected to dissect together, remind each other of what Galen had said about a particular structure and determine whether Galen was right.[31] As he fondly recalled, Vesalius himself had benefited from studying the structure of the larynx with a fellow student, Antonio Succha, a compatriot of 'rare promise in his remarkable knowledge of medicine and mathematics'.[32] Dissections became a collective activity of examining the body and comparing it with the text of Galen together. This, importantly, enabled Vesalius to call on those 'who have ever assisted me in dissection' to be witness to an anatomical fact – for example, that the liver was not divided into lobes.[33]

Vesalius's instruction on how to dissect the human body did not assume complete ignorance on the part of the student. He expected his students to be familiar with how the body was made and learn from images what to look for, so that they could dissect the body effectively. Dissection was a collective task where students reminded each other about the structure of the human body, helped each other in dissecting, and served as witnesses to what they saw or did not see.

THE MAKING AND UNMAKING OF THE HUMAN BODY

Knowledge of how the body was made thus relied on the unmaking of the body, and vice versa. That the processes of making and un-making were *both* necessary for understanding the human body was a point Vesalius made in striking terms with the construction of the articulated skeleton. For the purposes of studying bones, Vesalius acknowledged that having a collection of separate bones would be adequate.[34] Yet, he offered a lengthy instruction on how to construct a skeleton which was more suited to display in a public anatomy, as it could be compared with the body at the beginning of the dissection. Starting with an explanation of the bones was of course an important point of procedure for Vesalius in follow-ing the order in *On Anatomical Procedures*. The chapter (which was also the first printed account) on the construction of an articu-lated skeleton was one of the longest in *Fabrica*, and suggests that it mattered to Vesalius that he conveyed fully the details involved in making an articulated skeleton.

The process involved two stages – first obtaining bones from a cadaver and then putting the bones back together. To begin with, it was necessary to prepare a large cauldron like the one used by women in boiling lye. This could have evoked an association with the popular imagery of witches tending to their cauldrons, but Vesalius himself did not draw any explicit links.[35] Instead, he launched into detailed instructions. Remove from the cadaver the skin, muscles and organs, followed by the cartilages, the hyoid bone and the larynx (which are not to be boiled). Once all the bones are placed in the cauldron, pour in enough water so that the bones are covered at all times, and keep the liquid clear by removing the scum and fat that rise to the surface, as one normally does in cooking. No time is specified for the boiling as it depends on the size and age of the body. Pick out the bones with tongs and clean carefully, so as to keep the smooth cartilage with which bones are encrusted, but remove any flesh, ligaments or tendons.

Count the bones to check that all are present and immerse them in boiling fresh water. Rub them dry with a cloth, removing ligaments, membranes and insertions, but not the cartilage. Some of the bones could be placed around the fire to dry further, but not the breastbone, which should be cleaned carefully with a sprinkling of hot water and stored with its membrane in order to prevent it from twisting. The bones of the left and right arms, legs, toes and hands should be kept separately by wrapping them up in paper so that they do not get mixed up.

Vesalius was emphatic that the cleaning of bones should not be left to others with no experience or interest in anatomy, because it presented an opportunity to learn the texture and shape of the bones. He recalled his time in Paris at the Cemetery of Innocents,

> where we found a rich supply of bones, which we examined indefatigably over a long period until we were able to make a bet with our fellow-students that, blind-folded, we could identify by touch alone any bone which they pulled from the piles over a half-hour period and handed to us.[36]

Introduced as an example of the length to which he went to study the human body first-hand, this episode also served to demonstrate his manual mastery. It underscored the ability of the hand to distinguish and identify a bone by touch alone without the help of sight. This was a different kind of manual proficiency from the skill of dissecting that required careful viewing often guided by images. The work of cleaning and handling that could have been relegated to others because it was menial was now turned into an opportunity to acquire this tactile knowledge of bones.

If the seething of bones sounded like a cooking instruction, the next stage of assembling them into an upright skeleton read like a step-by-step manual for furniture assembly. Tools such as awls (like the ones for sewing soles onto shoes), copper wires

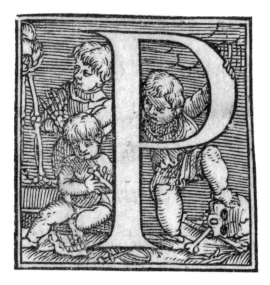

and forceps to bend and cut these wires were needed. The bones
were pierced by awls so that they could be joined together by
wires (coarse wires should be used for larger bones and finer ones
for smaller bones) using the techniques of 'repairing broken
plates and assembling stone cauldrons'. The skeleton was assembled from the feet up (illus. 70). First, the bones of the feet were
fastened onto a circular board. A hole was made near the edge
of the board for a rod that would take the weight of the skeleton. This rod could be in the shape of a spear, trident or scythe
(illus. 45). Another iron rod fixed on the circular board with
spikes was inserted through the foramen of the sacrum and the
vertebrae and bent to match the curve of the spine. The rod needed
to be longer than the skeleton so that it could be fixed to the
top of a box and enable rotation of the skeleton. The ribs could
be arranged in the correct order following the depressions for
the vein, nerve and artery, and by the fact that the upper part of
each rib is broader and denser than the one lower. But this was
fiddly work. Vesalius confessed that he had difficulty getting the

70 'The articulation of bones begins from the feet.' Woodcut 3.7 centimetres/
1½ in. square.

ribs connected in such a way as to show clearly 'the angle at which they naturally lie' because he left too large an interval between the top of the ilium and the tip of the twelfth thoracic rib.[37] Despite such difficulties, Vesalius thought that each person should do their best 'according to the diligence of his hand and his attention to what we have described so far in the entire book'.[38] Successful articulation of a skeleton was thus proof of one's manual dexterity *and* knowledge of the bones.

This process of breaking down the body to obtain the bones and then putting them back together to build a skeleton is akin to taking apart a clock and putting it back together. Taking apart a clock affords the opportunity to understand the parts that make up the clock, and putting the clock back together is confirmation of understanding how those parts fit together to make the clock. For Vesalius, this was achieved by the hand: knowing the human bones was tantamount to having the ability to make an articulated skeleton.

It is possible to make a case that something analogous was envisaged for the rest of the body with the paper manikins (illus. 56–9). While Vogtherr's printed flaps were sold ready-assembled (illus. 27), those in *Epitome* came with instructions on how to cut and construct them.[39] Readers were expected to cut out (probably with a knife) the printed nerves, veins, arteries and organs, having strengthened the paper with sturdier paper first. The copy of *Epitome* in Cambridge University Library shows a fourteenth-century legal manuscript recycled as backing material (illus. 4). The cut-outs had to be glued together correctly with the help of instructions and assembled into male and female figures. A certain amount of manual dexterity would have been needed to cut along the intricate course of blood vessels. In the absence of viable techniques for preserving the soft parts of the body in this period, a paper proxy was an artful way to incorporate in a book a process of manual construction.

We do not know to what extent readers of *Epitome* were successful in taking up Vesalius's invitation to use their hands to cut
out the paper parts of the body and assemble them into a layered
paper figure. Not many copies of *Epitome* have survived with the
manikins intact, and among the surviving ones, few have been cut
out so carefully as the copy at Cambridge. In contrast, we do know
that articulated skeletons became a vogue. In the seventeenth
century, the anatomical theatre at Leiden became a famous tourist
attraction for its display of skeletons of criminals and animals
holding banners of *memento mori*.[40]

Vesalius warned against those who believed that they could
learn how to sail from a book.[41] He did not expect his readers to
become proficient dissectors by simply reading or cutting pieces
of paper out of his books. It was nevertheless important for him
to convey the message by means of his book that both the making
and unmaking of the body were necessary to comprehend human
anatomy. This was also expressed in his instruction to the readers
of *Epitome* included at the foot of the title page (illus. 3): the book
could be read either from the beginning or from the end where
the male and female nudes were placed (illus. 53).

If beginning from the front of the book, the reader encountered
six brief chapters covering the whole of the body inside out,
starting with the bones. The text was followed by five full-size
muscle figures, abridged from *Fabrica*, beginning with the deepest
dissected figure numbered 'table five' (illus. 58). The subsequent
four figures (for example, illus. 35) were numbered in descending
order and with increasingly more muscles attached. The muscle
figures were followed by the figure of the skeleton leaning on the
sarcophagus from *Fabrica* (illus. 46), after which were placed the
male and female nudes surrounded by names of parts of the body
(illus. 53). The reverse numbering of the figures would have alerted
the reader starting from the beginning of the book that another
ordering was present in the book.

If starting from the nudes at the end of the book, the reader encountered a skeleton – just as Vesalius had brought in his articulated skeleton in his public anatomies. The reader then encountered the woodcuts of the muscles in ascending numerical order (and in increasing depth of dissection) towards the front of the book. The two directions of reading *Epitome* were another way to translate into the medium of the book the importance of the making *and* the unmaking of the human body.

We tend to associate anatomy with dissection and dismemberment which ends with the destruction of the human body. For Vesalius, however, human anatomy was as much about making the body as it was about unmaking it. This view shaped the content, arrangement and design of *Fabrica* and *Epitome*. He not only explained to his readers how to dissect a body and how to make a skeleton with their own hands, but also urged them to simulate the making of a body with the paper manikins. The ability to remake the body after its unmaking was proof of knowledge of the human body. It was akin to the power of the Creator of the *fabric* of the human body, to whom Vesalius points in the frontispiece (illus. 1).

IN MAKING HIS BOOK, Vesalius drew on all that his Renaissance world could offer – classical ideas, methods, tropes and sculptures; pictorial techniques of perspective and modelling; and the art of printing. And he drew on all his personal experience to date – in Louvain, Paris, Padua, Bologna and Venice. It was essential that Vesalius express his views of the body in a book, the emblem of learned physicians. It was only in a book that he could demonstrate his scholarly credentials and establish knowledge about the human body. But this book had to reflect his values also: explaining how the body was made depended on insights from first-hand dissection, and meaningful dissection presupposed knowledge of how the body was put together. This entailed the work of the hand with the quill as well as the knife. The hand, furthermore, had the ability to identify bones and remake them into a skeleton. The construction of the paper manikins simulated a similar work of the hand to make a paper body. The making and unmaking of the human body was a fitting design for a printed book created to convey the true knowledge of the human body. Ultimately, he hoped to convince the emperor that knowledge of human anatomy was fundamental to learned physicians, and that he – Vesalius – was the physician with that profound knowledge.

TEN

After *Fabrica*

ithin a month of the completion of printing in 1543, Vesalius presented lavishly coloured copies of *Fabrica* and *Epitome* to Charles V and was appointed one of his physicians.[1] His effort to get noticed in imperial circles with strategic publications and dedications that culminated in these two books had paid off. Vesalius then travelled back to Italy, going on what amounted to an exhibition tour of public anatomies or post-mortem dissections at Padua, Bologna, Pisa and Florence. He lingered in Florence, where he so impressed the Duke of Tuscany, Cosimo de' Medici, that Cosimo asked Charles V if he would release Vesalius from imperial service so that he could teach at the University of Pisa. Such a request no doubt made Vesalius all the more desirable as a physician to retain. The emperor refused to let him go.

LIFE AFTER *FABRICA*

Becoming an imperial physician meant joining a group of physicians, apothecaries, surgeons and other healers tasked to look after the health of the emperor and his household.[2] When Vesalius entered imperial service, the highest-ranking physician was Narciso Verdú of Naples (to whom he had dedicated his *Anatomical Tables* in 1538), who had been in post since 1524. Next in rank was Cornelis van Baersdorp, appointed slightly earlier than Vesalius in 1543. Both Verdú and Van Baersdorp were university-educated. Van Baersdorp may have descended from the Borsselen family with historically close connections to the dukes of Burgundy (the emperor's paternal ancestors), and had published a book summarizing the Galenic art of medicine (page height 29 centimetres/$11^2/5$ in., 180 pages), dedicated to the senate of Bruges and printed in Bruges.[3] Verdú, born in Naples, descended from an old Aragonese noble family, had not published any book, and appears to have treated his appointment as a sinecure as he rarely attended the court. When Verdú died, Van Baersdorp was expected to be promoted, but the emperor appointed another physician from Naples at the recommendation of the viceroy. Naples was a significant hereditary territory for Charles V as it gave him control of the southern half of the Italian peninsula. It is likely that political considerations affected some, if not all, appointments of this kind, since the physicians listed in the emperor's retinue in 1550 came from different parts of his territories. There was also Vesalius's mentor Nicolas Florenas, who was appointed imperial physician around 1530, probably through the influence of Johann van der Vort, physician to Margaret of Austria, governor of the Habsburg Netherlands and Charles V's aunt. Florenas seems to have moved to the court of Elector Frederick II and Dorothea of Denmark (the emperor's niece) in the early 1540s when he married his second wife, who was in Dorothea's service. To the consternation of the other imperial physicians, also at Charles V's court was one 'Dr Cavallus' of dubious credentials who nevertheless had Charles's ear as he offered advice that pleased the imperial patient who disliked restrictive treatments recommended by others for his gout. There were various ways of coming to the attention of the emperor.

In 1543, Verdú was in his early fifties and Van Baersdorp and Florenas were in their late fifties. Vesalius was not yet thirty years old. He was university-educated but did not hail from a famous family. There was no dramatic therapeutic or surgical feat that he could claim his own. Nor was he well connected with powerful elites who could put in a good word for him. Even with a family history in imperial service, for the son of an (illegitimate) apothecary to become an imperial physician demanded something striking that demonstrated his suitability for the post. A book was a hallmark of a learned physician. But by then, many had dedicated and published books to the great and the good in the hope of advancing their career. Catching the attention of an emperor therefore required something spectacular that stood out from the myriad of books churned out by university-educated physicians. It took something unusual and striking – something like *Fabrica*.

While *Fabrica* was an immediate success for Vesalius in his personal career, it did not change the world overnight. Galen's authority did not suffer a serious blow.[4] The *rete mirabile* did not swiftly disappear from the study of the human body.[5] For all the exhortation by Vesalius that public anatomies should be conducted differently, old habits died hard, even in Padua. After Vesalius's departure, a public anatomy was held in 1544. Realdo Colombo, who succeeded Vesalius as professor of surgery (for 70 florins a year), dissected the body, while da Monte, now the first ordinary professor of theory (for 700 florins a year), gave the anatomical explication, and Crassus, the second ordinary professor of practical medicine (for 200 florins a year) pointed out the relevant parts of the body.[6]

Nor did the book win instant approval from learned physicians. In particular, he found that people criticized his work to the emperor and other dignitaries. Determined never to write again, he burned his notes and the books of Galen he had studied and annotated – or at least that is what he said when, ironically, he took to the printed medium again. In 1546, Vesalius printed a letter addressed to an old friend, Joachim Roelants, then city physician of Mechlin, that ran to about two hundred pages (page

height *c.* 27 centimetres/10 ⅗ in.). It concerned the medicinal
efficacy of the 'China root' (*Smilax china* or *glabra*), which had re-
putedly helped the emperor's gout, but it was an opportunity for
Vesalius to defend himself against various critics of *Fabrica.*[7] Though
this publication on the China root was occasioned by the interest
of the imperial patient, Vesalius's knowledge of medicinal botany
was not confined to this substance. We know that he was also
familiar, for instance, with the use of guaiac wood (normally used
for treating syphilis) and sent a specimen of a 'true rhubarb' to
the professor of medicine at Tübingen, Leonhart Fuchs.[8] It is
nevertheless worth noting that when he chose to publish on thera-
peutics, it was in relation to his imperial patient, just as his other,
earlier book on treating 'pains of the side' was occasioned (as
Vesalius emphasized) by a personal interest of the emperor.

Vesalius accompanied Charles V on his campaigns across
Europe. In 1553, as they were leaving the camp at Mons in Hainaut
(about 50 kilometres/31 mi. southwest of Brussels), Vesalius met
one Abraham Ulrich, who was in the service of the Count of
Barby-Mühlingen.[9] He signed Ulrich's album with the same words
from his portrait, 'more swiftly, pleasantly and safely' (*ocyus, iucunde
et tuto*). It would have been an appropriate motto for an imperial
physician serving the emperor on a military campaign. We know
very little, however, about his work on the battlefield, other than
the fact that it did not impress the imperial surgeons.[10]

In 1555, a revised edition of *Fabrica* was printed by Oporinus.
The text was amended to include corrections and information
from additional dissections Vesalius had conducted. Some of the
woodcuts were corrected and revised, and surrounding areas of
some keyed letters were cut out to make them more visible. References to the individuals who had been cited in the first edition
to buttress Vesalius's views were dropped. He was now – as the
cartouche in the newly cut frontispiece announced – physician
(*medicus*) to the most invincible emperor (illus. 71).

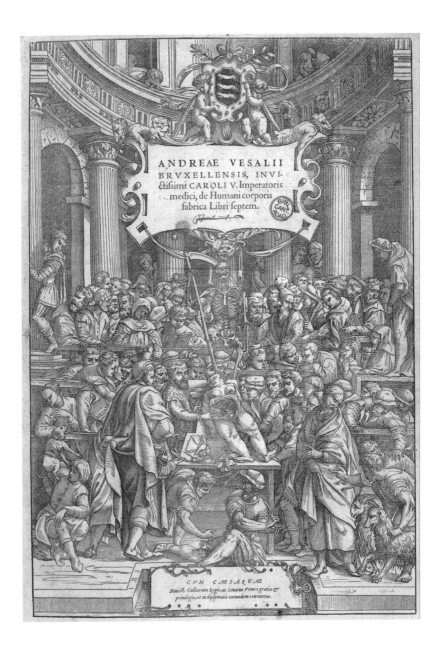

71 *Seven Books about the Fabric of the Human Body by Andreas Vesalius of Brussels, Physician to the Most Invincible Emperor, Charles V* (1555). Copy of Thomas Lorkyn (c. 1528–1591), Regius Professor of Physic in the University of Cambridge.

In his lifetime Vesalius's public fame rested largely on his *Fabrica* and the imperial appointment that the book had made possible. Like many learned physicians, Vesalius had published several other books before and since 1543, but none came close to *Fabrica* in size, complexity and ambition. This was the book that mattered to him most. He continued to annotate meticulously his own copy of the second edition. Perhaps he wanted to issue another edition, but if so, it did not materialize.[11]

When Charles V abdicated in 1556 in favour of his son, Philip II (the dedicatee of Vesalius's *Epitome*), he rewarded Vesalius as well as Van Baersdorp for their service by ennobling them. The charter of ennoblement for Vesalius singled out *Fabrica* as beyond compare in its eloquence, learning and usefulness, and 'easily and without question the greatest of all books which have been written about anatomy and celebrated for its illustrations'.[12] The book was indeed what distinguished Vesalius from the other physicians. By then, Charles had already parted with his copy of *Fabrica*, as he had given it to the French ambassador to the imperial court, Jacques Mesnage, soon after the cessation of war with France. While this might appear to be a sign that the emperor did not much care for Vesalius's book, it in fact underscores the book's value as an imperial object – beautifully coloured and bound in velvet – fitting for a diplomatic gift at a critical juncture of the empire's relations with France.[13]

After Charles's abdication, Vesalius moved to Philip's court in Madrid as physician to the courtiers from the Low Countries.[14] In 1559, Vesalius travelled at the behest of Philip to Paris when the French king Henri II (1519–1559) suffered a jousting injury to the head, which Ambroise Paré was also treating. In 1562, Vesalius was called to attend Don Carlos (1545–1568), Philip's son and heir, who suffered a head injury when he fell down the stairs. As was the custom at the time with serious royal injuries, Vesalius was but one among several other physicians, surgeons and sundry healers who were consulted by desperate family members who also prayed ardently for divine assistance. Vesalius's role in the death (in the case of Henri II) or survival (in the case of Don Carlos) of such royal patients is difficult to determine then or now. If he thought he had made any difference, he did not advertise it by publishing a book.

A few surviving medical opinions (*consilia*) offer a glimpse into Vesalius's practice as a physician.[15] Treatment for ailments such as weakening vision or epilepsy were determined on the premise that disease-causing humours needed to be rebalanced or evacuated. He wrote out recipes using plants and spices for medicinal drinks, syrups and pills; he prescribed regimens (for example, avoid intoxication and revelling; eat toasted bread, raisins or almonds); and he suggested surgical procedures such as bloodletting by cupping or leeches, cautery, or removal of suffusion in the eye with a needle. These were fairly common types of medical advice and the suggested surgical procedures were widely practised by surgeons at the time. They indicate a unified practice as a physician that Vesalius advocated in his address to the emperor in *Fabrica*. He also wanted his fellow physicians not to be afraid of surgery. When a former student, Giovanni Filippo Ingrassia, wrote to Vesalius about treating a fistula on the chest of the Marquis of Terranova dismissing the idea of surgery, Vesalius responded by explaining the anatomical details that justified surgery and his own success in treating similar cases.

In practice, Vesalius issued medical advice covering medication, regimen and surgery, though the kind of treatment offered was fairly conventional. His belief in the fundamental role of anatomical knowledge is reflected in his effort to ensure that his fellow physicians had sufficient anatomical knowledge to adopt surgical treatment where necessary. Vesalius offered and sometimes conducted surgical operations, but – as he noted – this went against the still prevailing expectation that physicians should not use their hands.[16]

While in Spain, Vesalius received a copy of *Anatomical Observations* (1561) by Gabriele Falloppio, professor of botany and surgery at Padua since 1551 (for two hundred florins a year).[17] Falloppio paid homage to the 'divine' Vesalius and his 'most perfect' work.[18] Having pursued 'truth' through extended efforts in dissection, he wrote that he had come to agree with most of what Vesalius had to say. Having found Vesalius's harsh criticism of Galen unbecoming of 'an anatomist, philosopher or physician', Falloppio was willing to credit others (including Berengario da Carpi and Ingrassia) with discoveries. Just as Vesalius criticized Galen as a follower of Galen, Falloppio presented himself as following Vesalius in correcting him. In the small booklet (page height *c.* 15.5 centimetres/6 in.) without illustrations, Falloppio listed his corrections or additions. He described, for example, for the first time the cochlea, the vestibular and tympanic ducts in the ear, the muscle lifting the eyelid (*musculus levator palpebrae*), and the extremity of the female seminal passage that resembled the bell of a brass trumpet (*tuba uterina*). Vesalius replied warmly at the end of 1561 from the 'Royal Court in Madrid', but the letter did not reach Falloppio before his untimely death. Although Vesalius objected to some of Falloppio's discoveries and crediting of others with discoveries, his emollient rhetoric probably helped Vesalius accept several of his findings. Vesalius was gratified that the professor of surgery at Padua, a position he once occupied, was adopting his method of following truth rather than authorities in dissection and supporting many (if not all) of his views.

Though Vesalius had published works framed as a (long) letter before, his letter to Falloppio seems not to have been intended for publication. According to the Venetian printer Francesco Franceschi, friends had urged Vesalius to publish it when he visited Francesco's shop in 1564 before setting off on a trip to the Holy Land. The booklet (page height *c.* 15 centimetres/6 in.), *A Consideration of Anatomical Observations by Falloppio* (1564), was published after

Vesalius had set sail. Vesalius had ended his letter to Falloppio expressing his hope that despite the difficulty of accessing bodies in Spain, he would at some point have the opportunity to scrutinize 'that true book of ours of the human body – man himself'.[19] These turned out to be his last words in print.

Vesalius travelled to Jerusalem and delivered a gift from Philip II to aid Catholic worshippers there. On the way back, he died on the Island of Zakynthos on 15 October 1564.

AFTERLIFE

Fabrica has continued to shape its author's reputation ever since. A recent worldwide census of *Fabrica* (both the 1543 and 1555 editions) helpfully illustrates its changing fortunes down to modern times.[20] Up to the year 1600, copies of *Fabrica* were owned by learned physicians, political elites and theologians. Not all owners inscribed their names or made annotations in their copies. Few readers read the book closely from cover to cover, line by line, image to image, correcting every single erratum. Readers were more likely to dip in and out of the parts they were interested in (which more often than not was the topic of the organs of generation). The book was certainly more comprehensive than its readers' immediate interests. Readers' notes, when present, reveal how *Fabrica* was read and what they brought to the reading of this book. Among its sixteenth-century readers was a student who had attended Vesalius's anatomy in Padua. More than ten years later, in his copy of the 1555 edition of *Fabrica*, this former student recalled his attendance at the famous university and recorded his personal connection to its (by then) famous former professor. The annotations also served to corroborate what Vesalius had written – just as he hoped that spectators in his theatre would.

Few readers of *Fabrica* commented specifically on the images, but the woodcuts certainly made an impression on some. Having

read *Fabrica* soon after its publication, one university-educated
annotator read Galen's *On the Usefulness of the Parts* in the most
up-to-date Latin translation in the edition overseen by da Monte
(1542).[21] In addition to jotting down in the margin noteworthy
points about the text, he made some drawings of what was discussed by Galen. For example, he drew a centaur where Galen
had cited Pindar on the question of why humans don't have
two hands and four legs like a centaur; where Galen remarked
that carnivores had claws for hunting and holding their prey, he
drew a bear clutching a bird. This reader who liked to annotate
pictorially then went to the trouble of neatly copying from *Fabrica*
images of the muscles of the arm and leg, the bones of the hand
and the facial muscles. The drawing of the arm (illus. 72) was
copied to indicate its three main parts (the upper arm, forearm
and hand) described by Galen, though the copying was detailed
enough to show other structures described in *Fabrica* (compare
illus. 38).[22] The other drawings copied from *Fabrica* were similarly
used to pick out fewer structures than Vesalius had indicated, and
focused on elucidating visually what Galen had written rather
than correcting or challenging Galen's words. It may appear odd
that images from a book that problematized the authority of
Galen would now be used to illustrate a work of Galen published
earlier. This example shows that *Fabrica*'s images achieved a status
as authoritative representations of the body itself and could be
copied without having to accept Vesalius's views.

By far the most significant impact of Vesalius's book was its
images. Rather than dismissing the phenomenon of copying as
rampant plagiarism by unscrupulous printers, it is worth noting
that it was also a process by which images of *Fabrica* became authoritative templates of the dissected human body.[23] Given the limited
availability and accessibility of a large, expensive book in Latin
that was *Fabrica*, it is through copied versions that Vesalius's work
reached a wider audience. The complex afterlife of *Fabrica*'s images

humidū uel paruum corpus continere conantur. Ad maiores enim moles uel fortiter comprehendendas & retinendas, uel fortiter emittēdas, æqualis undiꝗ comprehensio multum cōducit. Apparent uero in unam circuli circunferentiam conuenire digiti quinꝗ in actionibus huiusmodi, maxime quando exquisite sphæricum corpus comprehendunt. In his enim etiam manifestissime cognoscat aliquis id, quod in alijs quidē corporibus sit, non tamen æque apparet euidenter, quod digitorum summitates undiꝗ æqualiter oppositæ, tum suum ipsorum comprehensionem reddunt tutiorem & firmiorem, tum proiectiorem fortiorem edunt. Quemadmodū opinor, et in triremibus, remorum extremitates ad unam æqualitatem perueniunt, cum tamen ipsi omnes nō sint æquales. Et enim etiam ibi medios eandem ob causam maximos efficiūt. Ad manus autem claudendas, quando uel paruum corpus, uel humidum exacte uolumus continere, quod digitorum inæqualitas uti litatem præstat manifestissimā, id superiori sermone demōstratum esse arbitror, quo loco magnum digitum indici superuenientem, fieri uelut operculum superioris capacitatis, declarabam. In præsenti uero, dum adhuc pauca quædam adiecero, me totum ostendisse reor. Si enim in huiusmodi actionibus, interiorem digitum paruū longiorem factum esse intellexeris, aut aliquem mediorū breuiorem, aut oppositū eis magnum, aliam positionem uel magnitudinem habere, scies manifeste, quāto est optima præsens digitorū constitutio : quantumꝗ nocumenti sequetur actiones ipsas, siquid uel tantillum eorum, quæ ipsis insunt, transmutetur. Magna enim corpora, & parua, & siquid humidum comprehendere libet, non recte tractabimus, magnitudine alicuius digitorum immutata. Quō etiam manifestum est, quàm certa est præsens digitorum constructio. Primo huic libro finē imponere iam tempestiuū est. Reliquas enim totius manus particulas, & carpi, cubiti, brachij, libro secundo exponam. Deinde tertio, naturæ artem in cruribus ostendam. Quarto & quinto, nutriendi organa. Duobus uero sequētibus, de pulmone dicruribus. Octauo & nono, de ijs quæ ad caput pertinent. Solorum autem oculorum constructionem decimo exponam. Qui uero huic succedit liber, organa ad faciem attinentia continebit. Duodecimus, de ijs quæ dorsi sunt, exponet. Tertiusdecimus, quod erat reliquum, eorum quæ ad dorsum spectat, uel spatulas, id omnie adijciet. Duobus deinceps sequentibus, partes genitales, & ea quæ ad iꝗuꝗ, id est, coxæ uertebram attinent, declarabo. Sextusdecimus de cōmunibus animalis totius organis scilicet arterijs & uenis et neruis, sermonem faciet. Deinde, ueluti ἐπῳδόν aliquis post hos omnes, liber erit septimusdecimus, omnium particularum dispositionem simul cum proprijs magnitudinibus enarrans, demonstransꝗ totius operis utilitatem. *Galen.*

GALENI DE VSV PARTIVM CORPORIS HVMANI LIber secundus, Nicolao Regio Calabro interprete.

E usu partiū corporis humani scribere libro superiore aggressus, methodum primā declaraui : qua quis inueniat, in quam utilitatē unaquæque pars à natura sit creata. Narrationem uero à manu incepi, propterea quod hæc pars homini sit maxime propria. Deinceps hæc autem, cum omnes eius particulas ita persequi statuissem, ut ne minima quidem intētata relinqueretur: principio à digitis sermonem habui, quò demōstraui omnibus eorum particulis artem quandam mirabilem exprimi. Siquidem digitorum numerus, magnitudo, figura, cōstructioꝗ mutua, ad totius manus actionem, tam commode constituta ostendebatur, ut ne constructio quidē alia melior excogitari possit. Quoniam igitur liber primus in digitorum moribus finit, docuitꝗ primū uniuscuiusꝗ utilitatem: deinde autem duces eorum tendones, à musculis cubitū & radium circulo comprehendētibus, & à paruis summæ manus ortos: rationi consentaneum fuerit, etiam eorum quæ in hoc libro dicēda sunt, principium à musculorum narratione fecisse. Nam uniāquenꝗ eorum ita adornauit natura (quippe quem loco constituit idoneo, cuiꝗ originem tutissimā, & finem quò oportebat, produxit, & magnitudinem præstitit conuenientem, & securitatē, & numerum) ut ne constructio melior quidem excogitari queat. Mox enim, ut à multitudine incipiam (siquidē ubi quot cai, & quis motus cuiꝗ sit commissu, æquē erit utilitatem deinceps pertractare) numerus omniū cubiti, & manus extremæ musculorum, ad uiginti tres perueniēt: septem nāꝗ parui sunt in manu extrema: alij totidem magni totam interiorem cubiti regionem: reliqui nouem totam exteriorem occupauerūt. Parui itaꝗ manus extremæ musculi, duces sunt alterius obliquorū motuum. Eorum uero, qui tota intra cubitum, duo quidem maximi, digitos flectunt, magnitudine autem secundi duo etiam numero, totum carpum : obliqui uero duo, primum quidē radium, cum eo autem & totam manum ad pronā figuram circumagunt. Reliquus uero eorum septimus (qui minimus est eorum qui in longum extensi sint) ut quidem superiores anatomici putauerunt, flectit & ipse digitos quinqueꝗ:re uera autem, nullus motus alicuius digitorum ei commissus est, sed alterius cuiusdam mirabilis utilitatis gratia factus est, quam procedente sermone enarrabo. Ex his uero nouem musculis, qui in cubiti externa parte sunt, unus quidem digitos omnes, præterquam magnum extendit : duo uero alij eōdē quatuor digitos ad transuersum abducunt: quartus autem alius musculus solum magnum digitū mouet altero motu horum

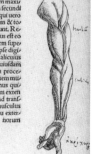

72 'The upper extremity consists of three main divisions, the upper arm, the forearm, and the hand.' Compare illus. 38. Galen, *On the Usefulness of the Parts* (1542). Page height 36.9 centimetres/ 14½ in.

can be illustrated by the three sets of engravings made within 25 years of *Fabrica*'s publication.

In the summer of 1544, Henry VIII, king of England, let it be known that he wanted *Fabrica*'s figures to be (re)published in England. According to Thomas Geminus (Lambrit), an instrument maker and engraver from Lixhe (north of Liége) working in London, Sir Anthony Denny had told him of the royal request just before the king left for the Siege of Boulogne.[24] Geminus obliged with a Latin tract, *Compendious Delineation of the Whole of Anatomy*, printed in 1545 and dedicated to the king. In the preface, Geminus noted how knowledge of anatomy was useful not only for physicians and surgeons, but also for those who wished to know about themselves and understand the greatest handiwork of the Creator. The book contained forty sheets of engravings, closely copying the woodcuts of *Fabrica* into a slightly smaller dimension (page height *c.* 38 centimetres/15 in.). While acknowledging Vesalius's expertise in anatomy, Geminus remarked that his prose was too prolix, and used instead the text of *Epitome*, which was printed with roman type in double columns in eighteen pages. Though Geminus copied from *Epitome* the large figures of the blood vessels and nerves as well as the nude figures somewhat altered (illus. 73), he did not copy the epitomized muscle figures (for example, illus. 35). In other words, *Fabrica*'s text was too long and *Epitome*'s images were too few. Denny rewarded Geminus with an annuity of £10 the year after this publication.

Geminus used his engravings in two more editions with an English text for the benefit of 'unlatined surgeons' as well as for those wishing to appreciate God's creation.[25] They were issued in 1553 and 1559 and dedicated to Edward VI and Elizabeth I respectively, with suitably adjusted title pages and prefaces. The English text, printed in Gothic type, is attributed to Thomas Vicary, surgeon to Edward VI and Elizabeth I, whom Geminus – himself a surgeon to Edward VI at one point – may also have known. It

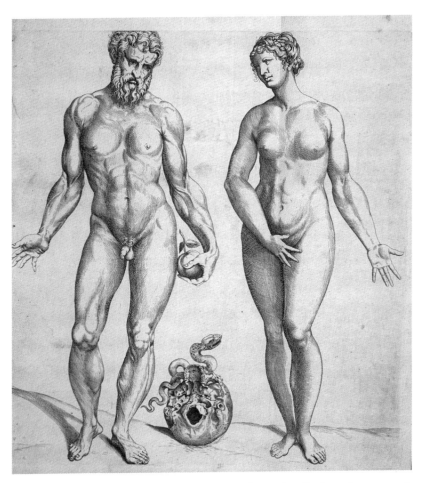

drew on material from Henry of Mondeville (*c.* 1260–*c.* 1320) and Lanfranc of Milan (1250–1306), and was arranged in the Mondinian order of dissection.[26] *Fabrica*'s images now illustrated a text for English surgeons derived from Mondino's time.

Geminus likely had contact with the humanist poet and physician Jacques Grévin when the latter visited England to avoid personal and religious troubles in France.[27] Geminus's printed

73 Engraving from Geminus, *Comependious Delineation* (1545). The apple, the skull and the serpent suggest the figures are of Adam and Eve (compare illus. 53). Page height *c.* 38 centimetres/15 in.

figures and plates migrated to Paris, where the printer André
Wechel issued a Latin edition, *Delineation of the Whole Anatomy*, in
1564, with the text of *Epitome* corrected by Grévin. Wechel was
no stranger to Vesalius's work, since he had printed earlier the
text of *Epitome* (1560) without the illustrations in a small format
(page height *c.* 18 centimetres/7 in.) at the behest of medical
students. The Greek words originally in the margins were moved
into the main Latin text so that students could use the margins
thus freed up to jot things down during a dissection.[28] Grévin's
edition of *Epitome* with Geminus's engravings was in a larger format
(page height *c.* 39 centimetres/15½ in.) with the text printed in
double columns in italic type. Grévin's comments were added
in roman type in a single column. Wechel dedicated this edition
to Count Philippe de Boulainvilliers Dammartin, Courtenay and
Fauquembergues, hoping that the book might help determine the
cause of a fever Philippe had been suffering for twelve years which
had confounded his physicians.[29] This was followed in 1569 by
Anatomical Portraits of All the Parts of the Human Body Engraved in Intaglio,
accompanied by a French translation of *Epitome* by Grévin.[30] With
this translation, Grévin hoped to aid those who were practising
medicine without the knowledge of Latin or Greek, so that French
careers could be built using French foundation stones, not 'por-
phyry from Greece or marble from Italy'. Geminus's images were
thus used to make available to those who could not access, afford
or read *Fabrica* a set of figures of the dissected human body which
were made comprehensible by an accompanying vernacular text.

Meanwhile, a second set of smaller engravings (page height
c. 29 centimetres/11⅖ in.) was made after the images in *Fabrica* to
accompany a Spanish text written by Juan Valverde of Hamusco,
A History of the Composition of the Human Body, for the benefit of Spanish
surgeons who did not know any Latin.[31] It was printed in Rome
in 1556 in roman type in a single column. Valverde dedicated the
book to Cardinal Juan Alvarez of Toledo, a powerful figure in the

Spanish community in Rome whom Valverde served as physician from 1555 after having served as assistant to Colombo. Because what Vesalius had written was difficult to understand without having seen the parts of the body first with the help of a good teacher, Valverde said that he had written briefly and concisely on what *he* had seen in bodies – he corrected, for example, the position of the lens in the eye from the centre towards the front of the eye. As for the images, Valverde had them mostly copied from *Fabrica*, though some of the images were altered (illus. 74). These were drawn by artists who were also patronized by Alvarez, Gaspar Becerra and possibly Pedro de Rubiales. Valverde explained that because his figures were engravings (and thus needed to be printed separately), they could not be 'mixed' with the text and so were put together at the end of each section. Valverde was explicit about the reason for copying: because *Fabrica*'s images were so well made, commissioning brand new images would have made Valverde appear jealous or mean-spirited; and the copied images indicated more easily where Valverde agreed or disagreed with Vesalius.[32] However, as he complained in the Italian translation of his work, *Anatomy of the Human Body*, issued in 1559, because he had copied Vesalius's images and because not many people understood Spanish, it was assumed that his work was just a translation of Vesalius's book.[33] He issued an Italian edition so that he could show his Italian gentlemen friends in Rome how his views were different from Vesalius's. At the same time, he refrained from producing a Latin edition, however, in deference to the publication *On Anatomical Matters* (1559) by his teacher, Colombo.[34] Although Valverde's differences with Vesalius as expressed in the modification of *Fabrica*'s images were comprehensible only to those who could read Spanish or Italian, his case of copying suggests that the images from Vesalius's book became equivalent in status to that of the 'canon' (Polycleitus' statue), against which others compared their own sculptures.

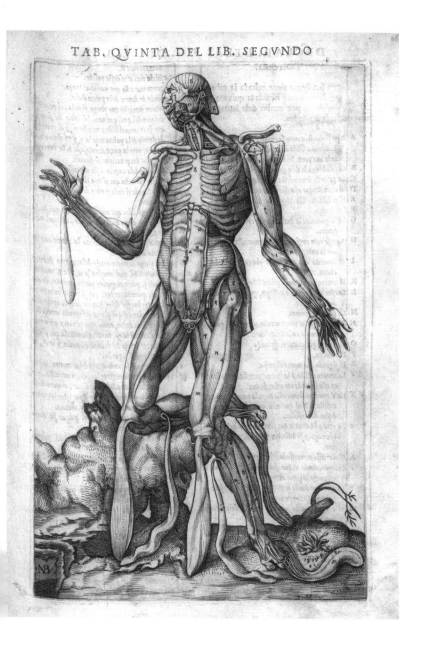

74 Nicolas Beatrizet's engraving for *A History of the Composition of the Human Body* (1556), copied from *Fabrica* (compare illus. 63) and modified to remove the animal muscles. Page height *c.* 29 centimetres/11²⁄₅ in.

The third case of copying was co-ordinated by the Antwerp publisher Christophe Plantin for a Latin book entitled *Lively Images of Parts of the Human Body Expressed in Copper*, printed in 1566 (page height *c.* 30 centimetres/11⁴⁄₅ in.).[35] The images were copied after Valverde's figures, engraved and printed by Pieter Huys with the help of his brother Frans. The legends for the figures were translated from Italian into Latin 'to assist all learned men'. Accompanying these images were the Latin text of *Epitome* as corrected by Grévin, and his comments, printed in italics. In short, Plantin had brought together a Latin edition derived from Vesalius's books once removed: the images (some of them revised) were copied from a book printed in Rome and the text with corrections was copied from a book published in Paris. In his dedication to the Antwerp Senate, Plantin defended his work as contributing to the good of the republic by publishing the best writings, including those that had been faultily printed before which were then corrected by learned men and printed by him with the most beautiful type. Acknowledging Vesalius's talent and erudition, Plantin declared that he published the book not to seek fame for himself, but to ensure that medical students would not be deprived of knowledge about the fabric of the human body.[36] He also promised a Dutch version, which was issued in 1568.

Given the expense – the cost of creating and printing engraved images was six times more than the expenditure on paper for Plantin (and much more expensive than woodcuts) – it is remarkable that *Fabrica*'s images were copied anew as engravings three times in the quarter-century after 1543. On each occasion, it was deemed worth the time, effort and cost to copy them. It is a compliment of sorts on the quality of the original woodcuts. Once created, printers optimized their use by issuing editions with text in different languages. The copied images could be paired with the text of *Epitome* (in Latin, sometimes corrected, or in French translation), an English text based on medieval works, or a Spanish

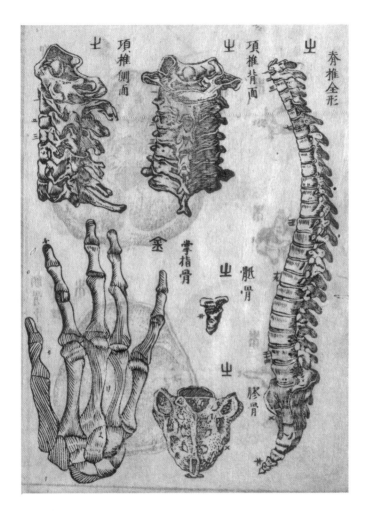

text of a contemporary physician or its Italian translation. They
were included in printed books, all smaller in size than *Fabrica* or
Epitome, addressing a variety of audiences who learned from these
images what a dissected human body looked like. Several other
publications in the period copied images from *Fabrica* less comprehensively, less well, in smaller dimensions and in woodcuts,

75 Sugita Genpaku, *Kaitaishinsho* (1774). Some of the woodcuts derive from
the Dutch version of *Vivae Imagines*. Page height 26 centimetres/10¼ in.

and paired them with different texts for different audiences. This kind of copying and recopying of images from *Fabrica* continued well beyond Vesalius's death and down the centuries. Recopied images several times removed from the original could be found as far as Edo-period Japan, for example (illus. 75).[37]

None of the publications that copied images from *Fabrica* were authorized by Vesalius. He took umbrage at the ones he knew about. We, too, may be disappointed that the images were almost immediately separated from the text, and the intricate relationship between text and image so carefully crafted by Vesalius was lost. Yet the examples above indicate that it was the copied images that enabled a range of people to engage with Vesalius's work in one way or another, directly or indirectly, even if it was in ways he had not envisaged or approved. The more these images were copied, the more people saw images that ultimately derived from *Fabrica*. The sum effect of frequent and active copying was that *Fabrica's* images became the most commonly available template for the dissected human body. But few copies were perfect facsimiles of the original woodcuts.[38] Just as artists added limbs to their sketches of the Belvedere Torso in emulation of an ancient masterpiece, images of *Fabrica* became models that could be altered and added to. Creative engagement of copying, modification and adjustment was what rendered *Fabrica's* images canonical.

It was people other than Vesalius – the readers, viewers, authors, printers, artists and others – who shaped the afterlife of *Fabrica*. Every generation brought to the book, or parts of the book, their own knowledge, expectations and hopes, and took away lessons and messages that made sense to them. They unmade and remade the book in their own image. In that process, Vesalius's own making and unmaking of the human body had largely dropped out of view.

CHRONOLOGY

1543	January: arrives in Basle
	May: dissects and makes an articulated skeleton of Jakob Karrer
	July: *Seven Books about the Fabric of the Human Body* and *Epitome of the Fabric of the Human Body* published in Basle by Johannes Oporinus
	August: German edition of *Fabrica*, translated by Albanus Torinus, printed in Basle by Oporinus
	August: presentation to Charles V of copies of *Fabrica* and *Epitome*, and appointment as imperial physician
1544	Anatomical demonstrations in Pisa at the invitation of Cosimo de' Medici
1544	Marries Anne van Hamme
1545	Daughter, Anne, born
1546	*Epistle Explaining the Method and Technique of Administering Boiled China Root which the Invincible Charles Recently Employed* printed in Basle by Oporinus
1555	Second edition of *Seven Books about the Fabric of the Human Body* printed in Basle by Oporinus
1556	Ennobled to Count Palatine by Charles V
	Abdication of Charles V, who cedes his Spanish territories to his son, Philip II
1559	Sent by Philip II to attend to the jousting injury of Henri II, King of France
1559	Moves to Philip's court in Madrid
1561	Receives a copy of *Anatomical Observations* by Gabriel Falloppio
1562	Tends to injury of Don Carlos, Philip's son
1564	*A Consideration of Anatomical Observations by Falloppio* printed in Venice by Francesco Franceschi
	March: journeys to the Holy Land and delivers Philip's gift to support Catholic worshippers in Jerusalem to the custodian of Holy Places
	15 October: dies on his way back to Europe on the Island of Zakynthos

REFERENCES

Abbreviations

Eriksson, *Eyewitness*   Ruben Eriksson, trans., *Andreas Vesalius'*
First Public Anatomy at Bologna 1540: An Eyewitness
Report by Baldasar Heseler (Uppsala and
Stockholm, 1959)

Fabrica   Andreas Vesalius, *De humani corporis fabrica*
(Basle, 1543)

Garrison and Hast   Daniel H. Garrison and Malcom H. Hast,
The Fabric of the Human Body: An Annotated
Translation of the 1543 and 1555 Editions of 'De
Humani Corporis Fabrica Libri Septem', 2 vols
(Basle, 2014)

O'Malley, *Vesalius*   Charles D. O'Malley, *Andreas Vesalius of*
Brussels, 1514–1564 (Berkeley, 1964)

Richardson and Carman   William Frank Richardson with John Burd
Carman, trans., *On the Fabric of the Human Body:*
A Translation of 'De Humani Corporis Fabrica Libri
Septem', 5 vols (San Francisco, 1998–2009)

Note: [ ] indicate the author's interpolation to clarify meanings, spell
out abbreviations, or supplement or correct paginations or foliations in the
original text.

Introduction

1 O'Malley, *Vesalius*, pp. 21–7.
2 *Fabrica*, fol.*2r; Garrison and Hast, vol. 1, p. 1 (cited).
3 Katharine Park, 'The Criminal and the Saintly Body: Autopsy and
Dissection in Renaissance Italy', *Renaissance Quarterly*, XLVII/1 (1994),
pp. 1–33, and other sources cited there.

4 Nancy G. Siraisi, *Medieval and Early Renaissance Medicine: An Introduction to Knowledge and Practice* (Chicago, IL, 1990), pp. 86–97.

5 This paragraph summarizes Vesalius's dedicatory letter to the emperor, *Fabrica*, fols *2r–*4v; Richardson and Carman, vol. I, p. I (cited).

6 Martin Davies, 'Humanism in Script and Print in the Fifteenth Century', in *The Cambridge Companion to Renaissance Humanism*, ed. Jill Kraye (Cambridge, 1996), pp. 47–62.

7 *Fabrica*, fol. *4v; Garrison and Hast, vol. I, p. 9 (cited) and n. 68.

8 For the recovery of classical remains and collections, see Kathleen Christian, *Empire without End: Antiquities Collections in Renaissance Rome, c. 1350–1527* (New Haven, CT, and London, 2010); Leonard Barkan, *Unearthing the Past: Archaeology and Aesthetics in the Making of Renaissance Culture* (New Haven, CT, and London, 1999); and Roberto Weiss, *The Renaissance Discovery of Classical Antiquity* (Oxford, 1969).

9 Tatjana Bartsch and Peter Seiler, eds, *Rom zeichnen: Maarten van Heemskerck 1532–1536/37* (Berlin, 2012); Phyllis Pray Bober and Ruth Rubinstein, *Renaissance Artists and Antique Sculpture*, 2nd edn (London, 2010), pp. 181–4.

10 See for example, Sebastiano Serlio, *On Architecture*, trans. Vaughan Hart, 2 vols (New Haven, CT, and London, 1996).

11 *Fabrica*, p. 548.

12 Many scholars have commented on the frontispiece: O'Malley, *Vesalius*, pp. 139–44; Andrew Cunningham, *The Anatomical Renaissance: The Resurrection of the Anatomical Projects of the Ancients* (Aldershot, 1997), pp. 124–8; Andrea Carlino, *Books of the Body: Anatomical Ritual and Renaissance Learning*, trans. John Tedeschi and Anne C. Tedeschi (Chicago, IL, 1999), pp. 43–52; Katharine Park, *Secrets of Women: Gender, Generation, and the Origins of Human Dissection* (New York, NY, 2006), pp. 207–49.

13 Ulinka Rublack, *Dressing Up: Cultural Identity in Renaissance Europe* (Oxford, 2010), pp. 51–6.

14 For the idea of artistic counterpoise, see David Summers, 'Contrapposto: Style and Meaning in Renaissance Art', *Art Bulletin*, LIX/3 (1977), pp. 336–61, esp. p. 343, n. 31.

15 *Fabrica*, p. 531; Garrison and Hast, vol. II, p. 1068 (cited). For mendicants' role in teaching theology at Padua, see Paul F. Grendler, *The Universities of the Italian Renaissance* (Baltimore, MD, 2002), pp. 357–72.

16 O'Malley, *Vesalius*, p. 142. For an overview of the history of eyeglasses, see Vincent Ilardi, *Renaissance Vision from Spectacles to*

Telescopes (Philadelphia, PA, 2007). I owe this reference to
  Professor Sven Dupré.
17 *Fabrica*, p. 655 (*specilli*); Garrison and Hast, vol. II, p. 1323 (cited).
18 Park, *Secrets of Women*, pp. 234–49.
19 Andreas Vesalius, *Epitome* (Basle, 1543), fol. Av. My translation.
20 Sachiko Kusukawa, *Picturing the Book of Nature: Image, Text, and
  Argument in Sixteenth-Century Human Anatomy and Medical Botany*
  (Chicago, IL, 2012), p. 200 (1 florin = 15 batzen).
21 Dániel Margócsy, Mark Somos and Stephen N. Joffe,
  *The Fabrica of Andreas Vesalius: A Worldwide Descriptive Census, Ownership,
  and Annotations of the 1543 and 1555 Editions* (Leiden, 2018),
  pp. 20–29.
22 Also noted in O'Malley, *Vesalius*, p. 142; Park, *Secrets of Women*,
  p. 256; Felix Platter, *Beloved Son Felix: The Journal of Felix Platter;
  A Medical Student in Montpellier in the Sixteenth Century*, trans. Seán
  Jennett (London, 1961), p. 47.
23 *Fabrica*, p. 76; Garrison and Hast, vol. I, pp. 153–4 (cited).

1 Learned Medicine and Its Books

1 Franz Fuchs, ed., *Hartmann Schedel (1440–1514): Leben und Werk*,
  Pirckheimer Jahrbuch für Renaissance- und Humanismusforschung,
  30 (Wiesbaden, 2016); Bettina Wagner, ed., *Worlds of Learning: The
  Library and World Chronicle of the Nuremberg Physician Hartmann Schedel
  (1440–1514)*, trans. Diane Booton and Bettina Wagner, exh. cat.,
  Bavarian State Library, Munich (2015).
2 Nancy G. Siraisi, 'The Faculty of Medicine', in *The History of the
  University in Europe*, vol. I: *Universities in the Middle Ages*, ed. H. de
  Ridder-Symoens (Cambridge, 1992), pp. 360–87.
3 Giovanna Pengo, ed., *Acta graduum academicorum gymnasii Patavini*,
  vol. II.2: *Ab anno 1461 ad annum 1470* (Padua, 1992), pp. 193–236.
4 Nancy G. Siraisi, *Medieval and Early Renaissance Medicine* (Chicago, IL,
  1990), pp. 58–77.
5 MS Clm 13, fol. 223r, Bavarian State Library, Munich. My translation
  and interpolation. The titles of books have been standardized and
  the names of professors follow the spelling in Tiziana Pesenti,
  *Professori e promotori di medicina nello studio di Padova dal 1405 al 1509:
  Repertorio bio-bibliografico* (Padua, 1984).
6 *Statuta almae universitatis d. artistarum, et medicorum Patavini gymnasii*
  (Venice, 1589), fols 38r, 68r–68v.

7 Nancy G. Siraisi, *Avicenna in Renaissance Italy: The Canon and Medical Teaching in Italian Universities after 1500* (Princeton, NJ, 1987), pp. 226–38; and Ian Maclean, *Logic, Signs and Nature: Learned Medicine in the Renaissance* (Cambridge, 2001), pp. 68–72.

8 *Statuta . . . Patavini gymnasii*, fol. 33v.

9 For the inferior status of surgery as an academic discipline, see Michael R. McVaugh, 'Surgical Education in the Middle Ages', *Dynamis*, XX (2000), pp. 283–304.

10 *Statuta . . . Patavini gymnasii*, fols 42r–v; translation at Jerome J. Bylebyl, 'Interpreting the *Fasciculo* Anatomy Scene', *Journal of the History of Medicine and Allied Sciences*, XLV/3 (1990), pp. 285–316, at p. 310.

11 'Anno D[omi]ni MccccLxv die xx marcij datu[s] fuit corpus pulc[her]ri[mu]m c[uius]dam vicentini a parente t[ame]n thetonicj: Rectori Odomatheo Padu[a]e[.] Celebraui[mus]q[ue] anothomiam [*sic*] e[ius] a die xx ad xxiiii diem e[ius]dem me[n]sis cu[m] summa vigilan[ti]a in pr[aesen]tia omn[ium] doctor[um] legentiu[m] n[e]cnon filij p[otes]tatis Anthonii bernardi utriusq[ue] iur[is] doctoris: Omniaq[ue] dubiola c[ir]c[a] corpus hu[m]anu[m] orie[n]tia p[er] doctores fuerunt disscussa [*sic*] at[que] tandem corp[us] cu[m] maxima festivitate humatu[m]: H[artmann] S[chedel].' MS Clm 363, fol. 186r, Bavarian State Library, Munich. My interpolations and translation. I thank Peter Jones and Lea Olsan for help with decoding Schedel's handwriting.

12 Andrea Carlino, *Books of the Body: Anatomical Ritual and Renaissance Learning*, trans. John Tedeschi and Anne C. Tedeschi (Chicago, IL, 1999), pp. 8–38.

13 *Statuta . . . Patavini gymnasii*, fol. 44v.

14 See, for example, Pesenti, *Professori e promotori di medicina*, pp. 42, 88–9, 137, 143, 185.

15 MS Clm 363, fol. 107r, Bavarian State Library, Munich; David S. Areford, *The Viewer and the Printed Image in Late Medieval Europe* (London, 2017), p. 109.

16 Jerome J. Bylebyl, 'The School of Padua: Humanistic Medicine in the Sixteenth Century', in *Health, Medicine and Mortality in the Sixteenth Century*, ed. Charles Webster (Cambridge, 1979), pp. 335–70, p. 339.

17 Paul F. Grendler, *The Universities of the Italian Renaissance* (Baltimore, MD, 2002), pp. 175–8.

18 Pengo, *Acta*, pp. 200–202.

19 Richard Palmer, *The 'Studio' of Venice and Its Graduates in the Sixteenth Century* (Padua, 1983), pp. 38–9.

20 Paul Fritz Joachimsen, ed., *Hermann Schedels Briefwechsel (1452–1478)*
    (Tübingen, 1893), nos 52, 55–7, pp. 106–113. Compare also David A.
    Lines, *The Dynamics of Learning in Early Modern Italy: Arts and Medicine at the
    University of Bologna* (Cambridge, MA, 2023), pp. 137–68; and
    Malcolm Parkes, 'The Provision of Books', in *The History of the
    University of Oxford*, vol. II: *Late Medieval Oxford*, ed. Jeremy Catto and
    Ralph Evans (Oxford, 1992), pp. 407–83. I thank Professor Teresa
    Webber for the last reference.

21 MS Clm 168, fol. 116v, Bavarian State Library, Munich.

22 Albert Derolez, *The Palaeography of Gothic Manuscript Books: From the
    Twelfth to the Early Sixteenth Century* (Cambridge, 2003), pp. 180–81;
    Henri-Jean Martin and Jean Vezin, eds, *Mise en page et mise en texte du
    livre manuscrit* (Paris, 1990).

23 Wagner, *Worlds of Learning*, pp. 34–62; Michail Chatzidakis, *Ciriaco
    d'Ancona und die Wiederentdeckung Griechenlands im 15. Jahrhundert*
    (Petersberg, 2017), pp. 331, 336–49, 356, 362, 426–37.

24 Debra Pincus, 'Calligraphy, Epigraphy, and the Paduan–
    Venetian Culture of Letters in the Early Renaissance', in *Padua
    and Venice: Transcultural Exchange in the Early Modern Age*, ed. Brigit
    Blass-Simmen and Stefan Weppelmann (Cambridge, 2017),
    pp. 41–60.

25 Davide Banzato Alberta de Nicolò Salmazo and Anna Maria
    Spiazzi, eds, *Mantegna e Padova 1445–1460*, exh. cat., Musei Eremitani,
    Milan (2006), pp. 62–79; Albinia C. de la Mare, Laura Nuvoloni
    and others, *Bartolomeo Sanvito: The Life and Work of a Renaissance Scribe*
    (Paris, 2009), pp. 129, 149, 385.

26 Martin Davies, 'Humanism in Script and Print in the Fifteenth
    Century', in *The Cambridge Companion to Renaissance Humanism*, ed. Jill
    Kraye (Cambridge, 1996), pp. 47–62, at p. 49.

27 See MS Clm 961, Bavarian State Library, Munich (Schedel's manual
    for constructing Greek and Latin letter forms); and Beatrice
    Hernad, *Die Graphiksammlung des Humanisten Hartmann Schedel*, exh. cat.,
    Bavarian State Library, Munich (1990), pp. 304–5. Schedel's new
    handwriting is characterized as a 'Gothic cursive-based all'antica
    book script' in Outi Merisalo, '*Scripsi manu mea*: Hartmann Schedel in
    Munich, Bayerische Staatsbibliothek, clm 490', *Ars et Humanitas*, VIII
    (2014), pp. 119–30, at p. 126.

28 Richard Stauber, *Die Schedelsche Bibliothek: Ein Beitrag zur Geschichte der
    Ausbreitung der italienischen Renaissance, des deutschen Humanismus und der
    medizinischen Literatur* (Nieuwkoop, 1969), pp. 52–101.

29 David McKitterick, *Print, Manuscript and the Search for Order, 1450–1830* (Cambridge, 2003), pp. 22–52.

30 Martin Lowry, *Nicholas Jenson and the Rise of Venetian Publishing in Renaissance Europe* (Blackwell, 1991), pp. 76–82, 137–72.

31 Areford, *The Viewer and the Printed Image*, pp. 105–63; Hernad, *Die Graphiksammlung*; McKitterick, *Search for Order*, pp. 53–96; compare Christopher Wood, *Forgery, Replica, Fiction: Temporalities of German Renaissance Art* (Chicago, IL, 2008), pp. 239–42.

32 For the conditions that governed learned book production, see Ian Maclean, 'The Diffusion of Learned Medicine in the Sixteenth Century through the Printed Book', in his *Learning and the Market Place: Essays in the History of the Early Modern Book* (Leiden, 2009), pp. 59–86, especially pp. 61, 67, 73.

33 Christian Coppens, '"For the Benefit of Ordinary People": The Dutch Translation of the *Fasciculus Medicinae*, Antwerp 1512', *Quaerendo*, XXXIX (2009), pp. 168–205, at pp. 199–203.

34 Bylebyl, 'Interpreting the *Fasciculo* Anatomy Scene', pp. 308–11; *Statuta . . . Patavini gymnasii*, fol. 42v (1465); Carlino, *Books of the Body*, pp. 9–20.

35 *Fabrica*, fol. *3r; Richardson and Carman, vol. I, p. li (cited).

36 Jeffrey Ashcroft, *Dürer: Documentary Biography* (New Haven, CT, and London, 2017), vol. I, pp. 45, 401–2 (93.5).

37 Klaus Arnold, 'Sebald Schreyer (1446–1520) als Kontrahent Hartmann Schedels, Förderer des Humanismus und der Sebaldverehurng in Nürnberg', in *Hartmann Schedel*, ed. Fuchs, pp. 145–211.

38 For the production process of this book, see Christoph Reske, *Die Produktion der Schedelschen Weltchronik in Nürnberg* (Wiesbaden, 2000), especially pp. 180–84.

39 Hartmann Schedel, *Liber chronicarum* (Nuremberg, 1493), fols 61r (Marseille), 110v (Metz), 194r (Nicea). Schedel's copy of *Liber chronicarum* at the Bavarian State Library, Munich, Rar.287, is digitized at www.digitale-sammlungen.de/view/bsb00034024.

2 Books and Careers

1 Ian Maclean, *Learning and the Market Place: Essays in the History of the Early Modern Book* (Leiden, 2009); Natalie Zemon Davis, 'Beyond the Market: Books as Gifts in Sixteenth-Century France', *Transactions of the Royal Historical Society*, 5th ser., XXXIII (1983), pp. 69–88.

2 For Aldus I follow Martin Lowry, *The World of Aldus Manutius: Business and Scholarship in Renaissance Venice* (Oxford, 1979) and Nicolas Barker, *Aldus Manutius and the Development of Greek Script and Type in the Fifteenth Century*, 2nd edn (New York, NY, 1992). Vivian Nutton, 'The Rise of Medical Humanism: Ferrara, 1464–1555', *Renaissance Studies*, XI/1 (1997), pp. 2–19.

3 N. Grant, ed. and trans., *Aldus Manutius: Humanism and the Latin Classics* (Cambridge, MA, 2017), p. 3.

4 N. G. Wilson, ed. and trans., *Aldus Manutius: The Greek Classics* (Cambridge, MA, 2016), p. 45.

5 The Greek version covers only up to part of Book Nine (on the brain), while the Arabic translation had preserved the entire book (to Book Fifteen), Charles Singer, trans., *Galen: On Anatomical Procedures*, repr. edn (Oxford, 1999), p. xxv.

6 Grant, *Manutius*, pp. 20–25, 242–5; Brian Richardson, '"Optimo Humanista et Greco": Aldus Manutius's Career in Venice in the Eyes of Marin Sanudo', *Erasmus Studies*, XXXV/2 (2015), pp. 181–209.

7 For Benedetti's biography, I follow Giovanna Ferrari, *L'Esperienza del passato: Alessandro Benedetti, filologo e medico umanista* (Florence, 1996), pp. 69–104.

8 Guido Ruggiero, 'The Status of Physicians and Surgeons in Renaissance Venice', *Journal of the History of Medicine and Allied Sciences*, XXXVI/2 (1981), pp. 168–84; Ferrari, *L'Esperienza del passato*, pp. 164–73.

9 Levi Robert Lind, *Studies in Pre-Vesalian Anatomy: Biography, Translations, Documents* (Philadelphia, PA, 1975), pp. 81–2 (cited).

10 Ibid., p. 83.

11 Ferrari, *L'Esperienza del passato*, pp. 161–2.

12 This paragraph summarizes Lind, *Pre-Vesalian Anatomy*, pp. 82, 84, 85, 91, 95, 103, 119–21, 124, 137.

13 Danielle Gourevitch, 'Le dossier philologique du nyctalope', in *Actes du Colloque hippocratique de Paris*, ed. Mirko D. Grmek (Paris, 1980), pp. 167–87.

14 Ferrari, *L'Esperienza del passato*, pp. 99–104.

15 For Berengario's biography, I follow Vittorio Putti, *Berengario da Carpi: Saggio biografico e bibliografico, seguito dalla traduzione del 'De fractura calvae sive cranei'* (Bologna, 1937), pp. 13–29.

16 Jacopo Berengario da Carpi, *Tractatus de fractura calve sive cranei* (Bologna, 1518), fol. XCr (*prudens medicus*); Levi Robert Lind, trans., *On Fracture of the Skull or Cranium by Berengario da Carpi* (Philadelphia, PA, 1990), p. 135 (cited in caption to illus. 15).

17 Lind, *On Fracture of the Skull*, p. 150.

18 For Berengario's *Commentary*, I follow Roger K. French, 'Berengario
    da Carpi and the Use of Commentary in Anatomical Teaching', in
    The Medical Renaissance of the Sixteenth Century, ed. Andrew Wear, Roger
    K. French and Iain M. Lonie (Cambridge, 1985), pp. 42–74. See also
    Andrea Carlino, *Books of the Body: Anatomical Ritual and Renaissance
    Learning*, trans. John Tedeschi and Anne C. Tedeschi (Chicago, IL,
    1999), p. 23, for the frontispiece.

19 Jacopo Berengario da Carpi, *Commentaria . . . super anatomia Mundini*
    (Bologna, 1521), fols LXXXVIIr, CCLXXIIr.

20 French, 'Berengario da Carpi', pp. 67–8.

21 Berengario, *Commentaria*, fols CVv, CLIIIr; Ian Maclean, *Logic, Signs and
    Nature: Learned Medicine in the Renaissance* (Cambridge, 2001),
    pp. 192–4.

22 In this paragraph, I summarize the points in Berengario,
    Commentaria, fols IIIIr [*sic*], VIr–VIIr, XXLIIIIr [*sic*], CXIXv, CXCIr
    (my emphasis added), CCXIv, CCXXIIv, CCLXr, CCXCVIIv, CCCIIIr,
    CCCCXXXVIIIr, CCCCXXXIXv, CCCCXLIv.

23 Ibid., fol. Lr.

24 Ibid., fol. CCCCLIXr–v.

25 Ibid., fols CCLXXIXr, CCCLXIIr.

26 Ibid., fols LXXVr, CCCCXLIIIIr [*sic*].

27 I have slightly modified the translation in Levi Robert Lind, trans.,
    A Short Introduction to Anatomy (Isagogae breves) (Chicago, IL, 1959),
    pp. 168 (cited in caption to illus. 17), 172 (for painters).

28 Berengario, *Commentaria*, fol. LXXXVIIr.

29 Putti, *Berengario*, pp. 194–9, suggests multiple hands in the design,
    including Ugo da Carpi; see Lind, *A Short Introduction*, pp. 26–7, for
    Rosso de Rossi.

30 Putti, *Berengario*, pp. 83–8, 116. See also the crucified figure at
    Berengario, *Commentaria*, fol. CCCCCXIXv.

31 Putti, *Berengario*, pp. 165–99.

32 Berengario being fifteen years senior to Alberto makes this
    statement more likely a literary licence on the part of Berengario
    about his time at Carpi. Putti, *Berengario*, pp. 13–14.

33 Stefania Fortuna, 'I Procedimenti Anatomici di Galeno e la
    traduzione Latina di Demetrio Calcondila', *Medicina nei Secoli*, XI/1
    (1999), pp. 9–28.

34 Vivian Nutton, '"Prisci Dissectionum Professores": Greek Texts and
    Renaissance Anatomists', in *The Uses of Greek and Latin: Historical Essays*,

ed. A. C. Dionisotti, Anthony Grafton and Jill Kraye (London, 1988), pp. 111–26, at pp. 114–15.

35 Charles Singer, trans., *Galen: On Anatomical Procedures*, repr. edn (Oxford, 1999), p. 2.

36 Galen, *Libri anatomici*, ed. Berengario da Carpi (Bologna, 1529), fols 3r–v.

37 Noted in Lind, *A Short Introduction*, p. 14.

38 Johannes Dryander, *Das Nocturnal* (Frankfurt am Main, 1535), fol. [Aij]r, *Novi Annuli* (Marburg, 1536), fols B[i]r–[Bii]v.

39 Albrecht Dürer, *Institutionum geometricarum libris* (Paris, 1532), p. 116.

40 D. H. Garrison, *Vesalius: The China Root Epistle: A New Translation and Critical Edition* (Cambridge, 2015), pp. 209–10.

41 Johannes Dryander, *Anatomia capitis* (Marburg, 1536), fol. [Aiij]r.

42 Eve M. Duffy and Alida C. Metcalf, *The Return of Hans Staden: A Go-Between in the Atlantic World* (Baltimore, MD, 2012), pp. 77–89.

43 For Massa, I follow Richard Palmer, 'Niccolò Massa, His Family, His Fortune', *Medical History*, XXV (1981), pp. 385–410, esp. pp. 403–5, for his finances.

44 Richard Palmer, *The 'Studio' of Venice and Its Graduates in the Sixteenth Century* (Padua, 1983), pp. 39–41.

45 This paragraph summarizes Lind, *Pre-Vesalian Anatomy*, pp. 174–7 (cited), 179–82, 203, 217, 241 (cited).

46 Niccolo Massa, *Liber introductorius anatomiae* (Venice, 1536), fol. 89v, as noted in Allen R. Shotwell, 'Dissection Techniques, Forensics and Anatomy in the 16th Century', in *The Body of Evidence: Corpses and Proofs in Early Modern European Medicine*, ed. Francesco Paolo de Ceglia (Leiden, 2020), pp. 107–18, at p. 118.

47 Miguel A. Granada and Dario Tessicini, 'Copernicus and Fracastoro: The Dedicatory Letters to Pope Paul III, the History of Astronomy, and the Quest for Patronage', *Studies in History and Philosophy of Science Part A*, XXXVI/3 (2005), pp. 431–76, at pp. 439–41.

48 Sarah Gwyneth Ross, *Everyday Renaissances: The Quest for Cultural Legitimacy in Venice* (Cambridge, MA, 2016), pp. 79–110. Nancy G. Siraisi, *Communities of Learned Experience: Epistolary Medicine in the Renaissance* (Baltimore, MD, 2013), pp. 17–20.

49 See, for example, other authors covered in Lind, *Pre-Vesalian Anatomy*.

3 Vesalius and the World of Books

1 For the biographical details, I follow O'Malley, *Vesalius*, pp. 23–7; Jacqueline Vons, trans., and Stéphane Velut, *Résumé de ses livres sur la fabrique du corps humain* (Paris, 2008), pp. VII–XXXVI.

2 Andrew Cunningham and Sachiko Kusukawa, *Natural Philosophy Epitomised: Books 8–11 of Gregor Reisch's Philosophical Pearl (1503)* (Aldershot, 2010), pp. 202–7.

3 For various images of the internal senses, see Edwin Clarke and Kenneth Dewhurst, *An Illustrated History of Brain Function* (Oxford, 1972).

4 *Fabrica*, p. 623; Garrison and Hast, vol. II, p. 1259 (cited in caption for illus. 20).

5 O'Malley, *Vesalius*, pp. 33–4; Henry de Vocht, ed., *Literae virorum eruditorum ad Franciscum Craneveldium 1522–1528*, Humanistica Lovaniensia, I (Louvain, 1928), p. 424.

6 *Fabrica*, fol. *3r; Richardson and Carman, vol. I, p. lii (cited).

7 O'Malley, *Vesalius*, p. 41.

8 Vivian Nutton, ed. and trans., *Principles of Anatomy according to the Opinion of Galen by Johann Guinter and Andreas Vesalius* (London, 2017), pp. 21–7.

9 Nutton, *Principles of Anatomy*, p. 66, n. 5.

10 *Fabrica*, p. 538.

11 Daniel H. Garrison, trans., *Vesalius: The China Root Epistle: A New Translation and Critical Edition* (New York, NY, 2015), p. 227 (cited); *Fabrica*, pp. 44 and 159, 511.

12 *Fabrica*, p. 498.

13 Hendrik D. Vervliet, *The Palaeotypography of the French Renaissance* (Leiden, 2008), vol. I, pp. 63–96, at p. 63 (cited).

14 Galen, *De anatomicis administrationibus libri novem*, trans. Johannes Guenther (Paris, 1531), fols [Aiij]v–[Aiv]v. Compare Aldus's edition of Niccolò Perotti, *Cornucopia* (1499), with consecutive numbering of lines in the internal margin, and the index using pagination and line number inserted before the main text.

15 Philippe Renouard, *Bibliographie des éditions de Simon de Colines, 1520–1546* (Paris, 1894), pp. 156–8, 180–81; Andrea Carlino, *Books of the Body: Anatomical Ritual and Renaissance Learning* (Chicago, IL, 1999), pp. 27–31.

16 Renouard, *Simon de Colines*, p. 264; Eugen A. Meier, M. Pfister-Burkhalter and Markus Schmid, *Andreas Cratander – Ein Basler Drucker und Verleger der Reformationszeit* (Basle, 1966), pp. 35–9; Vivian Nutton, 'Vesalius and His Publishers', in *La Fabrique de Vésale: La mémoire d'un livre*, ed. Jacqueline Vons (Paris, 2016), pp. 27–36, at p. 30.

17 Nutton, *Principles of Anatomy*, pp. 22–7.
18 As translated in Nutton, *Principles of Anatomy*, p. 89.
19 *Fabrica*, p. 161; Charles Singer, trans., *Galen: On Anatomical Procedures*, repr. edn (Oxford, 1999), p. 3.
20 O'Malley, *Vesalius*, p. 64.
21 'Rescius, Rutgerus', in *Contemporaries of Erasmus: A Biographical Register of the Renaissance and Reformation*, ed. Peter G. Bietenholz and Thomas Brian Deutscher (Toronto, 1985), vol. III, pp. 142–4.
22 Andreas Vesalius, *Paraphrasis* (Louvain, 1537), fols [2]r–5r.
23 O'Malley, *Vesalius*, pp. 25-6.
24 G. Baader, 'Jacques Dubois as a Practitioner', in *The Medical Renaissance of the Sixteenth Century*, ed. A. Wear, R. K. French and I. Lonie (Cambridge, 1985), pp. 146–54, at pp. 149–51.
25 Quintilian, *Institutio oratoria*, trans. H. E. Butler (London and New York, NY, 1921), vol. I, p. 157, vol. III, pp. 115–19.
26 As noted by Abdul Haq Compier, 'Rhazes in the Renaissance of Andreas Vesalius', *Medical History*, LVI/1 (2012), pp. 3–25, at pp. 10–12.
27 See, for example, Vesalius, *Paraphrasis*, fols 44r, 69r, 74r.
28 Vesalius, *Paraphrasis* (Basle, 1537); Nutton, *Principles of Anatomy*, pp. 7–8. I am grateful to Professor Nutton for sharing his latest analysis of the dating of this work.
29 Eckhard Kessler and Ian Maclean, eds, *Res et Verba in der Renaissance* (Wiesbaden, 2002).
30 Robert Zijlma and Tilman Falk, eds, *Hollstein's German Engravings, Etchings and Woodcuts 1400–1700*, vol. XIV B: *Hans Holbein the Younger* (Rosendaal, 1988), pp. 109–11 (no. 133).
31 Sachiko Kusukawa, 'Authority', in *A Cultural History of Medicine: The Renaissance*, ed. E. Leong and C. Stein (London, 2021), pp. 189–214, at pp. 195–6.
32 *Fabrica*, fol. *3r.
33 This paragraph and the next are indebted to Jerome J. Bylebyl, 'The School of Padua: Humanistic Medicine in the Sixteenth Century', in *Health, Medicine and Mortality in the Sixteenth Century*, ed. Charles Webster (Cambridge, 1979), pp. 335–70, esp. pp. 342–5.
34 Paul F. Grendler, *The Universities of the Italian Renaissance* (Baltimore, MD, 2002), pp. 21–34.
35 Jerry Stannard, 'Dioscorides', *Catalogus Translationum et Commentariorum*, IV (1980), pp. 1–144, at pp. 54–5 (Frigimelica); Theophilus Protospatharius, *De corporis humani fabrica libri quinque*, trans. Giunio Paolo Crasso (Venice, 1537).

36 E. Martellozzo Forin, ed., *Acta graduum academicorum gymnasii Patavini*, vol. III.3: *Ab anno 1538 ad annum 1550* (Padua, 1971), pp. 24–34; Richard Palmer, *The 'Studio' of Venice and Its Graduates in the Sixteenth Century* (Padua, 1983), pp. 31–4.

37 Jerome J. Bylebyl, 'The Manifest and the Hidden in the Renaissance Clinic', in *Medicine and the Five Senses*, ed. W. F. Bynum and Roy Porter (Cambridge, 1993), pp. 40–60. Note also Antonio Fracanzani's teaching at the hospital alongside da Monte. Michael Stolberg, 'Bedside Teaching and the Acquisition of Practical Skills in Mid-Sixteenth-Century Padua', *Journal of the History of Medicine and Allied Sciences*, LXIX/4 (2014), pp. 633–4.

38 Martellozzo Forin, ed., *Acta Graduum Academicorum Gymnasii Patavini*, vol. III.2. *Ab anno 1526 ad annum 1537* (Padua, 1970), pp. 447–8.

39 Jacobo Facciolati, ed., *Fasti gymnasii Patavini: Ab anno MDXVII ad MDCCLVI* (Padua, 1757), p. 385.

40 As a comparison, the rent of a student house (with four or five occupants) in Padua in the 1540s to 1560s averaged at about 20 florins a year: Grendler, *Renaissance Universities,* p. 167 (using conversation rate at p. 22, n. 55).

41 *Statuta almae universitatis d. artistarum et medicorum Patavini gymnasii* (Venice, 1589), fol. 33v.

42 Bylebyl, 'The School of Padua, p. 358.

43 Facciolati, *Fasti*, pp. 330–70; and Grendler, *Renaissance Universities,* p. 22, n. 55. Compare David A. Lines, *The Dynamics of Learning in Early Modern Italy: Arts and Medicine at the University of Bologna* (Cambridge, MA, 2023), pp. 51–3.

44 Bylebyl, 'The School of Padua', p. 344.

45 Facciolati, *Fasti*, p. 361 (Christophorus Sanctomaximus of Padua); Forin, *Acta* III.2, pp. 311–13.

46 Dagmar von Wille, 'Franciscus Frigimelica', *Dizionario biografico degli Italiani* (Rome, 1998), vol. L, pp. 538–40.

47 Nutton, *Principles of Anatomy*, pp. 27–36.

48 I follow Monique Kornell, 'Jan Steven van Calcar, *c.* 1515–*c.* 1546, Vesalius' Illustrator', in *Andreas Vesalius and the Fabrica in the Age of Printing: Art, Anatomy and Printing in the Italian Renaissance*, ed. Rinaldo F. Canalis and Massimo Ciavolella (Turnhout, 2018), pp. 99–130.

49 O'Malley, *Vesalius*, pp. 84, 431, n. 45.

50 *Fabrica*, fol. *4r; Richardson and Carman, vol. I, p. lvii (cited).

51 Facciolati, *Fasti*, p. 342; Vivian Nutton, '*Qui Magni Galeni Doctrinam in Re Medica Primus Revocavit*: Matteo Corti und der Galenismus im

medizinischen Unterricht in der Renaissance', in *Der Humanismus und die oberen Fakultäten*, ed. Gundolf Keil, Bernd Moelle and Winfried Trusen (Weinheim, 1987), pp. 173–84, at p. 173; Stefano Tomassetti, 'Benedetto Vittori', *Dizionario biografico degli Italiani* (Rome, 2020), vol. XCIX, pp. 829–31.

52 John M. Saunders and Charles Donald O'Malley, ed. and trans., *Andreas Vesalius Bruxellensis, The Bloodletting Letter of 1539: An Annotated Translation and Study of the Evolution of Vesalius's Scientific Development* (London, 1948).

53 O'Malley, *Vesalius*, p. 97.

54 Facciolati, *Fasti*, pp. 331, 343.

55 Andrea Carlino, 'Medical Humanism, Rhetoric, and Anatomy at Padua, circa 1540', in *Rhetoric and Medicine in Early Modern Europe*, ed. Stephen Pender and Nancy Struever (London, 2016), pp. 111–28, at pp. 121–3.

56 O'Malley, *Vesalius*, pp. 101–4; Vivian Nutton, ed. and trans., *An Autobibliography by John Caius* (Abingdon, 2018), pp. 58, 62–3.

57 *Fabrica*, p. 309; Richardson and Carman, vol. II, pp. 337–8 (cited).

4 The Making of the Book: The Printer and the Author

1 See Anja Wolkenhauer, *Zu schwer für Apoll: Die Antike in humanistischen Druckerzeichen des 16. Jahrhunderts* (Wiesbaden, 2002), pp. 384–96; for the sources and uses of the figure of Arion in the Renaissance, see K. Enenkel, *The Invention of the Emblem Book: Emblematization of Nature and the Poetics of Alciati's Epigrams* (Leiden, 2018), pp. 60–73.

2 Frank Muller, *Heinrich Vogtherr l'ancien: Un Artiste entre Renaissance et Réforme* (Wiesbaden, 1997), pp. 319–20 (no. 252).

3 Andrea Carlino, *Paper Bodies: A Catalogue of Anatomical Fugitive Sheets, 1538–1687*, trans. Noga Arikha (London, 1999), pp. 18–20 (no. 1); Muller, *Vogtherr l'ancien*, pp. 291–3 (no. 226). See also Suzanne Karr Schmidt, *Interactive and Sculptural Printmaking in the Renaissance* (Leiden, 2018), pp. 107–38.

4 Karr Schmidt, *Interactive and Sculptural Printmaking*, pp. 114–15.

5 Vivian Nutton, 'Vesalius and His Publishers', in *La Fabrique de Vésale: La mémoire d'un livre*, ed. Jacqueline Vons (Paris, 2016), pp. 27–36.

6 I follow Martin Steinmann, *Johannes Oporinus: Ein Basler Buchdrucker um die Mitte des 16 Jahrhunderts* (Basle and Stuttgart, 1967), pp. 1–19.

7 Oskar Bätschmann and Pascal Griener, *Hans Holbein* (London, 1999), p. 67; Frank Hieronymus, ed., *Basler Buchillustration 1500 bis 1545* (Basle, 1983), pp. xvi–xvii.

8 Christoph Reske, *Die Buchdrucker des 16. und 17. Jahrhunderts im deutschen Sprachgebiet: Auf der Grundlage des gleichnamigen Werkes von Josef Benzing* (Wiesbaden, 2007), pp. 78–80.

9 Bruce T. Moran, *Paracelsus: An Alchemical Life* (London, 2019), pp. 29, 95; Steinmann, *Oporinus,* p. 3.

10 Amy Nelson Burnett, 'The Reformation in Basel', in *A Companion to the Swiss Reformation*, ed. Amy Nelson Burnett and Emidio Campi (Leiden, 2016), pp. 170–215, at pp. 198–201; Steinmann, *Oporinus*, pp. 15–19.

11 Steinmann, *Oporinus*, p. 11. The business was not always amicable, however, as evidenced by a brawl between Lasius and Platter: Philip Gaskell, *A New Introduction to Bibliography*, repr. edn (Winchester, 1995), pp. 48–49.

12 Felix Platter, *Observationum . . . libri tres* (Basle, 1614), p. 11.

13 Harry Clark, 'The Publication of the Koran in Latin: A Reformation Dilemma', *Sixteenth Century Journal*, XV (1984), pp. 3–12; Steinmann, *Oporinus*, pp. 20–31.

14 As translated in Clark, 'Publication of the Koran', p. 9, my interpolation.

15 Steinmann, *Oporinus*, p. 12.

16 *Fabrica*, fol. [*5]r; Richardson and Carman, vol. I, p. lx (cited).

17 Martin Kemp, 'A Drawing for the *Fabrica*: And Some Thoughts upon the Vesalius Muscle-Men', *Medical History*, XIV (1970), pp. 277–88; William Breazeale, Cara Denison, Stacey Sell and Freyda Spira, *A Pioneering Collection: Master Drawings from the Crocker Art Museum* (London, 2010), pp. 58–60. A 'third' drawing of a skeleton, attributed to Calcar, offered for sale by Mattia Caiati (Milan) in 2019, has been established as of a later origin by Monique Kornell (personal communication).

18 Francis Ames-Lewis, *Drawing in Early Renaissance Italy*, 2nd edn (New Haven, CT, and London, 2000), pp. 55–6.

19 *Fabrica*, fol. [*5]r; Richardson and Carman, vol. I, p. lx (cited).

20 For the description of the woodblocks, I rely on Willy Wiegand, 'Marginal Notes by the Printer of the *Icones*', in S. W. Lambert, W. Wiegand and W. Ivins Jr, *Three Vesalian Essays to Accompany the Icones Anatomicae of 1934* (New York, NY, 1953), pp. 25–42.

21 O'Malley, *Vesalius*, p. 129.

22 Stoop went on to publish *Panygericum carmen* (1555) and *Poema* (1555); Bruce Nielsen, 'Daniel van Bombergen, a Bookman of Two Worlds', in *The Hebrew Book in Early Modern Italy*, ed. Joseph R. Hacker and Adam Shear (Philadelphia, PA, 2011), pp. 56–75.

23 O'Malley, *Vesalius*, pp. 183–7.

24 The italic type used in *Fabrica* is slightly larger than the roman type, which allows for a better balance between the letters and legibility, because the italic font is by default thinner and lighter than corresponding roman font, Roger Gaskell, 'The Typography and Layout of Vesalius's *De Fabrica* as specified in his Letter to Oporinus', *L'Illustrazione* III (2019), pp. 29–53. I am grateful to Mr Gaskell for sharing with me an earlier version of this paper.

25 Richardson and Carman, vol. II, p. xx.

26 *Fabrica*, fol. [*5]r; Richardson and Carman, vol. I, p. lix (cited).

27 *Fabrica*, pp. 306 [406]–310 [410] (pages in the 300s were misprinted; correct pages shown in square brackets).

28 This paragraph summarizes *Fabrica*, fol. [*5]r; Richardson and Carman, vol. I, p. lx (cited).

29 For example, *Fabrica*, pp. 172, 233 [333]. Compare the crisper printing of the woodblocks, see *Andreae Vesalii Bruxellensis Icones Anatomicae* (Munich, 1934 [1935]). I owe this observation to Professor Iain Donaldson.

30 Samuel W. Lambert, 'The Initial Letters of the Anatomical Treatise, *De humani corporis fabrica*, of Vesalius', in Lambert, Wiegand and Ivins, *Three Vesalian Essays*, pp. 3–24.

31 Allen R. Shotwell, 'The Revival of Vivisection in the Sixteenth Century', *Journal of the History of Biology*, XLVI/2 (2013), pp. 171–97, esp. pp. 180–89 for Vesalius.

32 *Fabrica*, p. 329 [429]; Garrison and Hast, vol. II, p. 867 (cited in caption to illus. 31).

33 Alexander Marr, 'Walther Ryff, Plagiarism and Imitation in Sixteenth-Century Germany', *Print Quarterly*, XXXI/2 (2014), pp. 131–43.

34 *Fabrica*, p. 267 [367]; Richardson and Carman, vol. III, p. 31.

35 *Fabrica*, fol. Kk2v; Nutton, 'Vesalius and His Publishers', pp. 33–4. See also Vesalius's correction of the second edition: Vivian Nutton, 'Vesalius Revised: His Annotations to the 1555 *Fabrica*', *Medical History*, LVI/4 (2012), pp. 415–43.

36 O'Malley, *Vesalius*, p. 136.

37 *Fabrica*, fols Kk3r–[Mm3]v.

38 I owe this observation to Dániel Margócsy.

39 *Fabrica*, fol. Ll2r; Richardson and Carman, vol. V, pp. 300–301 (cited in caption for illus. 34).

40 *Fabrica*, fol. Kk3r.

41 Ian Maclean, *Logic, Signs and Nature: Learned Medicine in the Renaissance* (Cambridge, 2001), p. 59.

42 *Fabrica*, pp. 203, 206, 208, 609, 610, 611.

43 Steinmann, *Oporinus*, pp. 45–7, 60–71.

5 The Human Figure: Art and Anatomy

1 Eriksson, *Eyewitness*, p. 139, my interpolation.

2 Joanna Woods-Marsden, *Renaissance Self-Portraiture: The Visual Construction of Identity and the Social Status of the Artist* (New Haven, CT, and London, 1998); Machtelt Israëls, *Piero Della Francesca and the Invention of the Artist* (London, 2021).

3 Anthony Grafton, *Leon Battista Alberti: Master Builder of the Italian Renaissance* (London, 2001); and Leon Battista Alberti, *On Painting and On Sculpture*, trans. Cecil Grayson (London, 1972).

4 Alberti, *On Painting*, pp. 75, 85; Alberti, *On Sculpture*, pp. 138–9.

5 Alberti, *On Painting*, p. 75.

6 Ibid., p. 99.

7 Here I follow Alison Wright, *The Pollaiuolo Brothers: The Arts of Florence and Rome* (New Haven, CT, and London, 2005), pp. 158–65.

8 Eckart Marchand, 'Plaster and Plaster Casts in Renaissance Italy', in *Plaster Casts: Making, Collecting, and Displaying from Classical Antiquity to the Present*, ed. Rune Frederiksen and Eckart Marchand (Berlin, 2010), pp. 49–79. For the role of casts in achieving lifelikeness, see Fredrika Herman Jacobs, *The Living Image in Renaissance Art* (Cambridge, 2005), pp. 176–85.

9 Paula Findlen, et al., *Leonardo's Library: The World of a Renaissance Reader*, exh. cat., Stanford University, Stanford, CA (2019), pp. 5–15. For Leonardo, I follow Martin Kemp, *Leonardo da Vinci: The Marvellous Works of Nature and Man*, revd edn (Oxford, 2006), pp. 10–21.

10 Kemp, *Leonardo da Vinci*, pp. 250–52.

11 Monica Azzolini, 'Leonardo da Vinci's Anatomical Studies in Milan: A Re-Examination of Sites and Sources', in *Visualizing Medieval Medicine and Natural History, 1200–1550*, ed. Jean A. Givens, Karen Reeds and Alain Touwaide (Aldershot, 2006), pp. 147–76, at pp. 161–2.

12 Martin Clayton and Ron Philo, eds, *Leonardo da Vinci: Anatomist* (Royal Collections, 2012), nos 25–31, 47–8, 52–4, 58–9, 83.

13 Alessandro Nova, '"La Dolce Morte": Die anatomischen Zeichnungen Leonardo da Vincis als Erkenntnismittel und reflektierte Kunstpraxis', in *Zergliederungen: Anatomie und Wahrnehmung in der frühen*

Neuzeit, ed. Albert Schirrmeister and Mathias Pozsgai (Frankfurt am Main, 2005), pp. 136–63; Alessandro Nova and Domenico Laurenza, eds, *Leonardo da Vinci's Anatomical World* (Venice, 2011).

14 Nancy G. Siraisi, *The Clock and the Mirror: Girolamo Cardano and Renaissance Medicine* (Princeton, NJ, 1997), p. 110.

15 A. Aymonino, 'Nature Perfected: The Theory and Practice of Drawing after the Antique', in *Drawn from the Antique: Artists and the Classical Ideal*, ed. A. Aymonino and A. Lauder, exh. cat., Teylers Museum, Haarlem, and Sir John Soane's Museum, London (London, 2015), pp. 15–67; Ernst Gombrich, 'The Style all'antica: Imitation and Assimilation', in his *Norm and Form: Studies in the Art of the Renaissance* (London, 1966), pp. 22–8.

16 James Elkins, 'Michelangelo and the Human Form: His Knowledge and Use of Anatomy', *Art History*, VII/2 (1984), pp. 176–86, at p. 181.

17 Rocco Sinisgalli, *Leon Battista Alberti, On Painting: A New Translation and Critical Edition* (Cambridge, 2011), pp. 4–6.

18 *Fabrica*, p. 171; Richardson and Carman, vol. II, p. 5 (cited in caption to illus. 38, my insertion).

19 *Fabrica*, p. 175; Richardson and Carman, vol. II, pp. 13–14 (cited in caption to illus. 39, my insertion).

20 Monique Kornell, 'Jan Steven van Calcar, c. 1515–c. 1546, Vesalius' Illustrator', in *Andreas Vesalius and the Fabrica in the Age of Printing: Art, Anatomy and Printing in the Italian Renaissance*, ed. Rinaldo F. Canalis and Massimo Ciavolella (Turnhout, 2018), pp. 99–130.

21 Martin Kemp, 'A Drawing for the *Fabrica*: And Some Thoughts upon the Vesalius Muscle-Men', *Medical History*, XIV (1970), pp. 277–88, at pp. 285–6. For Campagnola's prints, see David Rosand and M. Murano, eds, *Titian and the Venetian Woodcut*, exh. cat. National Gallery Washington (1976), pp. 120–37, 154–65.

22 Giulio Bodon, *Heroum Imagines: La Sala dei Giganti a Padova; Un monumento della tradizione classica e della cultura antiquaria* (Venice, 2009).

23 Patricia Simons and Monique Kornell, 'Annibal Caro's After-Dinner Speech (1536) and the Question of Titian as Vesalius's Illustrator', *Renaissance Quarterly*, LXI/4 (2008), pp. 1069–97.

24 Willy Wiegand, 'Marginal Notes by the Printer of the Icones', in S. W. Lambert, W. Wiegand and W. Ivins Jr, *Three Vesalian Essays to accompany the Icones Anatomicae of 1934* (New York, 1953), pp. 25–42.

25 Francisco Guerra, 'The Identity of the Artists Involved in Vesalius's Fabrica 1543', *Medical History*, XIII (1969), pp. 37–50; Rosand and Murano, *Titian and the Venetian Woodcut*.

26 Daniel H. Garrison, trans., *Vesalius: The China Root Epistle: A New Translation and Critical Edition* (Cambridge, 2015), p. 227.

27 *Fabrica*, fol. *4r.

28 *Fabrica*, p. 195; Richardson and Carman, vol. II, p. 60 (cited in caption to illus. 40).

29 For example, *Fabrica*, pp. 376–7 [476–7], 560–61.

30 *Fabrica*, p. 263 [363]; Garrison and Hast, vol. II, p. 712 (cited in caption to illus. 41, my insertion).

31 *Fabrica*, p. 180; Garrison and Hast, vol. II, p. 357 (cited in caption to illus. 42, my insertions).

32 As noted in Glenn Harcourt, 'Andreas Vesalius and the Anatomy of Antique Sculpture', *Representations*, XVII (1987), pp. 28–61, at pp. 32–4.

33 *Fabrica*, p. 160; Richardson and Carman, vol. I, p. 380 (cited in caption to illus. 45).

34 *Fabrica*, p. 12, Garrison and Hast, vol. I, p. 32, n. 9.

35 *Fabrica*, p. 164; Richardson and Carman, vol. I, p. 388 (cited in caption to illus. 46).

36 *Fabrica*, fol. *2r. Compare Viktoria von Hoffmann, 'Ingeniosa Peritia: The Language of Ingenuity in Italian Renaissance Anatomy', in *Ingenuity in the Making: Matter and Technique in Early Modern Europe*, ed. Richard J. Oosterhoff, José Ramón Marcaida and Alexander Marr (Pittsburgh, PA, 2021), pp. 94–111, at pp. 102–3.

37 *Fabrica*, fol. *2v. Pliny the Elder, *Natural History*, trans. H. Rackham, W.H.S. Jones and D. E. Eichholz (London, 1938), vol. V, pp. 26–7.

38 *Fabrica*, pp. 260–61, 242, 309; Richardson and Carman, vol. II, pp. 214, 168, 337 (cited).

39 Jacqueline Vons and Stéphane Velut, *Résumé de ses livres sur la fabrique du corps* (Paris, 2008), p. lxviii.

40 Dániel Margócsy, Mark Somos and Stephen N. Joffe, eds, *The Fabrica of Andreas Vesalius: A Worldwide Descriptive Census, Ownership, and Annotations of the 1543 and 1555 Editions* (Leiden, 2018), pp. 81, 215. See also Paul Reichel, *Tödlein Schrein* (c. 1580), Kunsthistorisches Museum, Vienna, Austria (Kunstkammer, 4450).

41 Rose Marie San Juan, 'The Turn of the Skull: Andreas Vesalius and the Early Modern Memento Mori', *Art History*, XXXV/5 (2012), pp. 958–75, at pp. 969–70.

42 Wiegand, 'Marginal Notes', pp. 39–41.

43 Ulinka Rublack, ed., *The Dance of Death by Hans Holbein* (London, 2016).

44 *Fabrica*, p. 169; Richardson and Carman, vol. II, pp. 1–2 (cited).

45 Harcourt, 'Anatomy of Antique Sculpture', p. 30; Monique Kornell,
    Erin Travers, Thisbe Gensler and Naoko Takahatake, *Flesh and Bones:
    The Art of Anatomy*, exh. cat. Getty Museum, Los Angeles (2022),
    pp. 35–8.
46 Vivian Nutton, *Principles of Anatomy according to the Opinion of Galen by
    Johann Guinter and Andreas Vesalius* (London, 2017), p. 103, n. 61.
47 *Fabrica*, p. 592; Garrison and Hast, vol. II, p. 1198 (cited).
48 *Fabrica*, p. 268.
49 Ibid., pp. 94, 127, 559, 599.
50 Ibid., pp. 150, 271, 294, 300, 305, 335–6 [435–6], my translation.
51 Ibid., p. 610 (at YY).
52 Ibid., pp. 62, 227 [327] (not repeating images); repeated woodcuts at
    pp. 22 and 38, 36 and 47.
53 For example, ibid., p. 336 [436] (at T).

6 Theatre

 1 *Fabrica*, p. 548.
 2 Eriksson, *Eyewitness*, pp. 85–7, 306–7.
 3 E. Martellozzo Forin, ed., *Acta graduum academicorum gymnasii Patavini*,
    vol. III.2: *Ab anno 1526 ad annum 1537* (Padua, 1970), pp. 447–8.
 4 Ibid., vol. III.3: *Ab anno 1538 ad annum 1550* (Padua, 1971), pp. 5, 7, 14, 23,
    34, 51, 57, 67, 69, 70.
 5 O'Malley, *Vesalius*, pp. 78-9.
 6 Eriksson, *Eyewitness*, p. 139.
 7 Angelo Ventura, 'Marcantonio Contarini', in *Dizionario Biografico degli
    Italiani*, ed. Alberto Maria Ghisalberti and M. Pavan (Rome, 1983),
    vol. XXVIII, pp. 237–41.
 8 *Fabrica*, pp. 650–51; Garrison and Hast, vol. II, p. 1315 (cited).
 9 *Fabrica*, p. 162; Garrison and Hast, vol. I, p. 314 (cited); O'Malley,
    Vesalius, p. 64.
10 For the various criminal punishments in Venice, see *Leggi criminali del
    Serenissimo Dominio Veneto* (Venice, 1751).
11 *Fabrica*, p. 248 [348]; Garrison and Hast, vol. I, p. 679 (cited).
12 Joel F. Harrington, *The Faithful Executioner: Life and Death in the Sixteenth
    Century* (London, 2014), pp. 185–225.
13 *Fabrica*, p. 324 [424]; Richardson and Carman, vol. III, p. 184.
14 *Fabrica*, pp. 584–5; Garrison and Hast, vol. II, pp. 1183–4 (cited).
15 Andrea Carlino, *Books of the Body: Anatomical Ritual and Renaissance
    Learning*, trans. John Tedeschi and Anne C. Tedeschi (Chicago, IL,

1999), pp. 118–19. Note, however, the later association of public anatomies as continuation of criminal punishment: Anuradha Gobin, *Picturing Punishment: The Spectacle and Material Afterlife of the Criminal Body in the Dutch Republic* (Toronto, 2021), p. 142. I thank Dániel Margócsy for drawing my attention to the latter book.

16 *Fabrica*, p. 245.

17 Ibid., p. 561; Richardson and Carman, vol. v, p. 4 (cited in caption to illus. 50).

18 *Statuta almae universtitatis d. artistarum et medicorum Patavini gymnasii* (Venice, 1589), fol. 67v; Katharine Park, 'The Criminal and the Saintly Body: Autopsy and Dissection in Renaissance Italy', *Renaissance Quarterly*, XLVII/1 (1994), pp. 1–33, at p. 12.

19 *Fabrica*, p. 512. For a similar case, see Cynthia Klestinec, *Theaters of Anatomy: Students, Teachers, and Traditions of Dissection in Renaissance Venice* (Baltimore, MD, 2011), pp. 127–8.

20 *Fabrica*, p. 512; Garrison and Hast, vol. II, p. 1032.

21 *Fabrica*, pp. 324 [424], 377 [477], 510, 538–9.

22 Paul F. Grendler, *The Roman Inquisition and the Venetian Press 1540–1605* (Princeton, NJ, 1977), p. 207.

23 For the populations of Padua and Venice around this time, respectively, see Paul F. Grendler, *The Universities of the Italian Renaissance* (Baltimore, MD, 2002), p. 38; and David Chambers, Brian S. Pullan and Jennifer Fletcher, eds, *Venice: A Documentary History 1450–1630* (Oxford, 1992), p. 107.

24 *Fabrica*, pp. 495, 512, 538, 540, 585. See also M. Biesbrouck and O. Steeno, 'Andreas Vesalius's Corpses', *Acta Medico-Historica Adriatica*, XII/1 (2014), pp. 9–26, at pp. 25–6.

25 *Fabrica*, pp. 538–9; Garrison and Hast, vol. II, p. 1081 (cited).

26 Massimo Galtarossa, 'Knowledge from Bodies and Resistance to Anatomical Discourse (Padua, 16th–18th Centuries)', in *The Body of Evidence: Corpses and Proofs in Early Modern European Medicine*, ed. Francesco Paolo de Ceglia (Leiden, 2020), pp. 175–90, at p. 177.

27 For these arrangements, see *Statuta . . . Patavini gymnasii*, fols 27v–28r, 42r.

28 My translation from A. Germain, *La Renaissance à Montpellier: Étude historique d'après les documents originaux avec pièces justificatives inédites* (Montpellier, 1871), pp. 151–2; also as already noted in Karl H. Dannenfeldt, *Leonhard Rauwolf: Sixteenth-Century Physician, Botanist, and Traveler* (Cambridge, MA, 1999), pp. 24–5.

29 Nicholas Terpstra, 'Piety and Punishment: The Lay Conforteria and
    Civic Justice in Sixteenth-Century Bologna', *Sixteenth Century Journal*
    XXII/4 (1991), pp. 679–94, at p. 685, n. 28; Eriksson, *Eyewitness*,
    p. 223; Carlino, *Books of the Body*, pp. 109–15.

30 Nicholas Terpstra, 'Confraternities and Capital Punishment: Charity,
    Culture, and Civic Religion in the Communal and Confessional Age',
    in *A Companion to Medieval and Early Modern Confraternities*, ed. Konrad
    Eisenbichler (Leiden, 2019), pp. 212–31, at p. 214.

31 As noted in Katharine Park, *Secrets of Women: Gender, Generation, and the
    Origins of Human Dissection* (New York, 2006), pp. 212–13, 216–17.

32 *Fabrica*, pp. 551, 553.

33 Grendler, *Renaissance Universities*, p. 34. See also the caution expressed
    in David A. Lines, *The Dynamics of Learning in Early Modern Italy: Arts and
    Medicine at the University of Bologna* (Cambridge, MA, 2023), pp. 44–8.

34 Estimate based on Forin, *Acta*, vol. III.2 (1526–1537), pp. 377–450,
    vol. III.3 (1538–1550), pp. 3–89.

35 Jacopo Berengario, *Commentaria . . . super anatomia Mundini* (Bologna,
    1521), fol. CCXXIIv.

36 Eriksson, *Eyewitness*, pp. 85–7.

37 *Fabrica* (1555), p. 681; Garrison and Hast, vol. II, p. 1134 (cited).

38 Park, 'The Criminal and Saintly Body', p. 15.

39 *Statuta . . . Patavini gymnasii*, fol. 42v.

40 *Fabrica*, p. 279 [379]; Garrison and Hast, vol. II, p. 747 (cited).

41 *Fabrica*, p. 547.

42 Eriksson, *Eyewitness*, p. 109 (cited), 149 (Leipzig).

43 Ibid., pp. 247 and 293 (cited).

44 *Fabrica*, p. 222 [322]; Richardson and Carman, vol. II, p. 373 (cited).

45 Eriksson, *Eyewitness*, pp. 221, 287. For tighter control of student
    behaviour at Padua later in the century, see Cynthia Klestinec,
    'Civility, Comportment, and the Anatomy Theater: Girolamo
    Fabrici and His Medical Students in Renaissance Padua', *Renaissance
    Quarterly*, LX/2 (2007), pp. 434–63.

46 *Fabrica*, p. 279 [379].

47 A. Germain, 'Les Étudiants de l'école de medicine de Montpellier au
    XVIe siècle étude historique sur le liber procuratoris studiosorum',
    Revue historique, III (1877), pp. 31–77, at p. 61.

48 O'Malley, *Vesalius*, pp. 79–80; MS Clm 363, fol. 186r, Bavarian State
    Library, Munich.

49 O'Malley, *Vesalius*, pp. 137–8. Karrer's skeleton articulated by Vesalius
    survives at the Anatomical Museum at Basle.

50 *Fabrica*, p. 548.

51 Ibid., pp. 548–58, 603, 656.

52 Eriksson, *Eyewitness*, p. 227.

53 Ibid., pp. 219, 227, 253, 283. See also Charles D. O'Malley, 'The Anatomical Sketches of Vitus Tritonius Athesinus and Their Relationship to Vesalius' *Tabulae Anatomicae*', *Journal of the History of Medicine and Allied Sciences*, XIII/3 (1958), 395–97.

54 *Fabrica*, p. 659 [663]; Garrison and Hast, vol. II, 1337 (cited).

55 R. Allen Shotwell, 'Animals, Pictures, and Skeletons: Andreas Vesalius's Reinvention of the Public Anatomy Lesson', *Journal of the History of Medicine and Allied Sciences*, LXXI/1 (2016), pp. 1–18.

56 For the separation of the anatomy lectures in the 1520s, see Jerome J. Bylebyl, 'The School of Padua: Humanistic Medicine in the Sixteenth Century', in *Health, Medicine and Mortality in the Sixteenth Century*, ed. Charles Webster (Cambridge, 1979), pp. 335–70, at p. 356.

57 Eriksson, *Eyewitness*, pp. 47–9. For Corti, see Vivian Nutton, '*Qui Magni Galeni Doctrinam in Re Medica Primus Revocavit*: Matteo Corti und der Galenismus im medizinischen Unterricht in der Renaissance', in *Der Humanismus und die oberen Fakultäten*, ed. Gundolf Keil, Bernd Moelle and Winfried Trusen (Weinheim, 1987), pp. 173–84.

58 *Fabrica*, p. 547.

59 This spat is noted by Andrew Cunningham, *The Anatomical Renaissance: The Resurrection of the Anatomical Projects of the Ancients* (Aldershot, 1997), pp. 110–13; Eriksson, *Eyewitness*, p. 273.

7 The Bodies in the Book

1 *Fabrica*, fol. *3v.

2 Ibid., pp. 280 [380], 548.

3 Nancy G. Siraisi, 'Vesalius and Human Diversity in *De Humani Corporis Fabrica*', *Journal of the Warburg and Courtauld Institutes*, LVII (1994), pp. 60–88; Glenn Harcourt, 'Andreas Vesalius and the Anatomy of Antique Sculpture', *Representations*, XVII (1987), pp. 28–61.

4 *Fabrica*, p. 529; Richardson and Carman, vol. IV, p. 167 (cited).

5 *Fabrica*, p. 585.

6 Ibid., p. 89.

7 Nancy G. Siraisi, 'Vesalius and the Reading of Galen's Teleology', *Renaissance Quarterly*, L/1 (1997), pp. 1–37.

8 William L. Straus Jr, and Owsei Temkin, 'Vesalius and the Problem of
   Variability', *Bulletin of the History of Medicine*, XIV/5 (1943), pp. 609–33;
   Fabrica, pp. 52, 119; Richardson and Carman, vol. I, p. 279 (cited in
   caption for illus. 54).

9 Wilhelm Pfitzner, 'Beiträge zur Kenntnis des menschlichen
   Extremitätenskelets', *Morphologischen Arbeiten*, IV/3 (1895), pp. 347–
   570, at pp. 543 4; Wenzel Gruber, 'Ungewöhnliches Ossiculum
   Sesamoideum am Handrucken', *Archiv für Anatomie, Physiologie und
   wissenschaftlicher Medicin* (1870), pp. 499–500.

10 Hippolyte Cloquet, *Traité d'anatomie descriptive,* 3rd edn (Paris, 1824),
   p. 103, no. 224; Henry Gray, *Anatomy, Descriptive and Surgical* (London,
   1858), pp. 33, 57.

11 Alexander Macalister, with Alexander Carte, 'On the Anatomy of
   Balænoptera Rostrata', *Philosophical Transactions of the Royal Society,*
   CLVIII (1868), pp. 201–61 at p. 208; *Text-Book of Human Anatomy*
   (London, 1889), p. 534; Dániel Margócsy, Mark Somos and Stephen
   N. Joffe, *The Fabrica of Andreas Vesalius: A Worldwide Descriptive Census,
   Ownership, and Annotations of the 1543 and 1555 Editions* (Leiden, 2018),
   pp. 222–3.

12 This paragraph is based on *Fabrica*, pp. 17–19; Garrison and Hast,
   vol. I, p. 45 (cited in caption for illus. 55, my interpolation; I have
   also modifed the translation).

13 For the separation of pathology from anatomy, see Siraisi, 'Vesalius
   and Human Diversity', pp. 81–3.

14 *Fabrica*, pp. 242, 529; 'Claudius de Simeonibus Utinensis' received a
   doctorate in law in 1540; E. Martellozzo Forin, ed., *Acta graduum
   academicorum gymnasii Patavini*, vol. III.3: *Ab anno 1538 ad annum 1550*
   (Padua, 1971), pp. 61–2.

15 *Fabrica*, p. 124; Richardson and Carman, vol. I, p. 292 (cited);
   Garrison and Hast, vol. I, p. 241, n. 44 (Marfan's syndrome). Angelo
   M. G. Scorza, *Le famiglie nobili genovesi* (Genova, 2009), p. 65.

16 See, for example, James G. Harper, ed., *The Turk and Islam in the Western
   Eye, 1450–1750: Visual Imagery before Orientalism* (Farnham, 2011).

17 *Fabrica*, p. 248.

18 Ibid., pp. 230 [330], 253 [353]; Richardson and Carman, vol. II,
   p. 394 (cited); see also O'Malley, *Vesalius*, pp. 114–17.

19 *Fabrica*, p. 292.

20 Ibid., p. 348 [448]; Garrison and Hast, vol. II, p. 906 (cited).

21 *Fabrica*, p. 252 [352]. This notation for the dance position 'twice
   simple' appears to have been fairly common. See *L'Art et instruction de*

bien dancer (Paris, 1495, facsimile 1936); and Thoinot Arbeau,
Orchésographie (Langres, 1589), fol. 40r.

22 *Fabrica*, p. 46.
23 Ibid., p. 390 [490].
24 Ibid., pp. 353–4 [453–4].
25 Ibid., p. 536; Richardson and Carman vol. IV, p. 182 (cited).
26 *Epitome*, fol. Fv. Captions to illus. 56–59 are my translation.
27 *Fabrica*, p. 520; Richardson and Carman, vol. IV, p. 145 (cited).
28 *Fabrica*, p. 521; Richardson and Carman, vol. IV, p. 146 (cited).
29 Katharine Park, *Secrets of Women: Gender, Generation, and the Origins of
    Human Dissection* (New York, 2006), pp. 218–19.
30 *Fabrica*, p. 383 [483]; Richardson and Carman, vol. IV, p. 48 (cited).
31 *Fabrica*, p. 543; Richardson and Carman, vol. IV, p. 200 (cited).
32 *Fabrica*, pp. 373–4 [472–4], 379–80 [479–80]; Garrison and Hast,
    vol. II, p. 966 (cited in caption to illus. 60); Harcourt, 'Anatomy of
    Antique Sculpture', p. 30.
33 As acknowledged in *Fabrica*, p. 303.
34 Ibid., pp. 374 [474], 522–6; Garrison and Hast, vol. II, p. 958 (cited).
    Compare Margaret Tallmadge May, trans., *Galen: On the Usefulness of the
    Parts of the Body* (Ithaca, NY, 1968), vol. II, pp. 635–6, for Galen's
    theory of sex determination.
35 *Fabrica*, p. 537.
36 Ibid., p. 525; Garrison and Hast, vol. II, pp. 1057–8 (cited).
37 *Fabrica*, p. 545. See also Vivian Nutton, *Ancient Medicine* (London,
    2004), p. 235.
38 Park, *Secrets of Women*, pp. 219–20.
39 *Fabrica*, p. 533; Richardson and Carman, vol. IV, p. 176 (cited).
40 *Fabrica*, p. 381 [481]; Garrison and Hast, vol. II, p. 970 (cited in
    caption to illus. 61).
41 Thomas Laqueur, *Making Sex: Body and Gender from the Greeks to Freud*
    (Cambridge, MA, 1990), pp. 81–3; against which, see Katharine
    Park, 'The Myth of the "One-Sex" Body', *Isis*, CXIV/1 (2023),
    pp. 150–75; and Helen King, *The One-Sex Body on Trial: The Classical
    and Early Modern Evidence* (Farnham, 2013), pp. 13–17, 49–70.
42 *Fabrica*, pp. 36, 46, 56, 131, 313.
43 Gianna Pomata, 'Menstruating Men: Similarity and Difference of
    the Sexes in Early Modern Medicine', in *Generation and Degeneration*,
    ed. Valeria Finucci and Kevin Brownlee (Durham, NC, 2001),
    pp. 109–52, at pp. 111–12; and Vivian Nutton, 'Montanus, Vesalius
    and the Haemorrhoidal Veins', *Clio Medica*, XVIII (1983), pp. 33–6.

44 O'Malley, *Vesalius*, pp. 150–81.
45 *Fabrica*, pp. 244 [344], 255 [355].
46 Ibid., p. 500.
47 Ibid., p. 36; Richardson and Carman, vol. I, p. 89 (cited in caption to illus. 62).
48 *Fabrica*, pp. 186, 288; Garrison and Hast, vol. I, pp. 373 (cited in caption to illus. 63), 572.
49 Charles Singer, trans., *Galen: On Anatomical Procedures*, repr. edn (Oxford, 1999), pp. 76–7.
50 R. Allen Shotwell, 'Animals, Pictures, and Skeletons: Andreas Vesalius's Reinvention of the Public Anatomy Lesson', *Journal of the History of Medicine and Allied Sciences*, LXXI/I (2016), pp. 1–18. See also *Fabrica*, p. 162.
51 *Fabrica*, pp. 55, 295 [395], 382 [482]; and following J. B. de C. M. Saunders and Charles D. O'Malley, *The Anatomical Drawings of Andreas Vesalius* (New York, NY, 1982), pp. 61, 136; Richardson and Carman, vol. II, p. xix.
52 *Fabrica*, p. 589.
53 Ibid, pp. 145, 231 [331], 255 [355], 282 [382], 310 [410], 500, 545, 648; Letizia Panizza, 'The Semantic Field of "Paradox" in 16th and 17th Century Italy: From Truth in Appearance False to Falsehood in Appearance True; A Preliminary Investigation', in *Il vocabolario della république des lettres*, ed. M. Fattori (Florence, 1997), pp. 197–220; Agnieszka Steczowicz, '"The Defence of Contraries": Paradox in the Late Renaissance Disciplines', DPhil thesis, Oxford University (2004), pp. 149–79.
54 *Fabrica*, p. 600; Garrison and Hast, vol. II, p. 1214 (cited).

8 Vesalius: Surgeon, Anatomist, Physician?

1 This paragraph summarizes the preface, *Fabrica*, fols *2r–*3r; Richardson and Carman, vol. I, pp. xlix–liii (cited).
2 *Fabrica*, p. 494.
3 Ibid., pp. 30, 199, 234, 245; Richardson and Carman, vol. II, p. 68 (cited).
4 *Fabrica*, p. 30; Richardson and Carman, vol. I, p. 70 (cited in caption to illus. 65).
5 Margaret Tallmadge May, trans., *Galen: On the Usefulness of the Parts of the Body* (Ithaca, NY, 1968), vol. I, pp. 364–5.
6 *Fabrica*, p. 660.

7 Ibid., p. 237 [235].
8 Ibid., pp. 239, 553, 601, 603.
9 Ibid., p. 236, and for his use of instruments, see for example, ibid., pp. 238, 261, 269–70, 293.
10 For example, ibid., pp. 238, 269–70, 293, 552, 601.
11 Ibid., pp. 234, 260, 267, 222 [322], 226 [326], 255 [355].
12 Ibid., p. 236 [336], 549.
13 Ibid., pp. 552, 603; Garrison and Hast, vol. II, 1121 (cited).
14 *Fabrica*, pp. 278, 214 [314], 516.
15 Ibid., p. 651; Garrison and Hast, vol. II, p. 1315–16 (cited in caption for illus. 67).
16 *Fabrica*, p. 237.
17 Ibid., pp. 277 [377].
18 Ibid., fol. Kk3r (index), referring to pp. 94, 390 [490], 391 [491], 392 [492], 500, 590. For other occurrences of *anatomici*, see, for example, pp. 118, 142, 221, 307, 220 [320], 234 [334], 535; *professores dissectionum*, pp. 10, 100, 246, 270, 277; *professores anatomes*, pp. 10, 82, 154, 312.
19 Ibid., fol. *3r (*prisci professores dissectionum*), pp. 270, 300, 245 [345]; Vivian Nutton, '"Prisci Dissectionum Professores": Greek Texts and Renaissance Anatomists', in *The Uses of Greek and Latin: Historical Essays*, ed. A. C. Dionisotti, Anthony Grafton and Jill Kraye (London, 1988), pp. 111–26, at pp. 116–17.
20 *Fabrica*, pp. 218 [318], 591.
21 See, for example, ibid., p. 391 [491].
22 This paragraph summarizes the points made ibid., pp. 83, 276 [376], 282 [382]; Richardson and Carman, vol. I, p. 194; Garrison and Hast, vol. II, pp. 741, 750 (cited).
23 I follow here the discussion by Andrew Cunningham, *The Anatomical Renaissance: The Resurrection of the Anatomical Projects of the Ancients* (Aldershot, 1997), pp. 103–13, 226–7.
24 Eriksson, *Eyewitness*, pp. 84–5, 306, n. 12.
25 Ibid., pp. 44–7.
26 Ibid., p. 289.
27 *Fabrica*, p. 642; Garrison and Hast, vol. II, p. 1299. My emphasis.
28 *Fabrica*, p. 643.
29 Gianna Pomata, 'A Word of the Empirics: The Ancient Concept of Observation and Its Recovery in Early Modern Medicine', *Annals of Science*, LXVIII (2011), pp. 1–25.
30 *Fabrica*, pp. 43, 55, 98, 154–5, 309.

31 This paragraph summarizes ibid., pp. 216–17[316–17], 219 [319], 227 [327].
32 Ibid., p. 125–6; Garrison and Hast, vol. I, p. 249, n. 11.
33 *Fabrica*, p. 594; Richardson and Carman, vol. v, pp. 92–3 (cited).
34 *Fabrica*, pp. 594–9.
35 Ibid., pp. 622–4.
36 Ibid., p. 636.
37 Cunningham, *The Anatomical Renaissance*, pp. 88–142.
38 *Fabrica*, p. 591.
39 Ibid., p. 237 [337]; Richardson and Carman, vol. II, p. 410 (cited).
40 *Fabrica*, p. 83.
41 Ibid., p. 521; Garrison and Hast, vol. II, pp. 1050 (cited). Other references to the same phrase are at *Fabrica*, pp. 65, 538, 591.
42 Horace, *Epistles*, 1.14, in Horace, *Satires, Epistles, The Art of Poetry*, trans. H. Rushton Fairclough (Cambridge, MA, 1978), pp. 251–3.
43 For the adoption of this motto by the Royal Society, see Michael Hunter, *Establishing the New Science: The Experience of the Early Royal Society* (Woodbridge, 1989), pp. 1–43.
44 Ian Maclean, *Logic, Signs and Nature: Learned Medicine in the Renaissance* (Cambridge, 2001), pp. 192–4.
45 *Fabrica*, fol. *3v, pp. 82–3, 218 [318].
46 Monique Kornell, 'Jan Steven van Calcar, c. 1515–c. 1546, Vesalius' Illustrator', in *Andreas Vesalius and the Fabrica in the Age of Printing: Art, Anatomy and Printing in the Italian Renaissance*, ed. Rinaldo F. Canalis and Massimo Ciavolella (Turnhout, 2018), pp. 99–130, at p. 119.
47 *Fabrica*, p. 223 [323]; Garrison and Hast, vol. I, pp. 633–4 (cited).
48 O'Malley, *Vesalius*, p. 148.
49 *Fabrica*, p. 306; Richardson and Carman, vol. II, p. 331 (cited).
50 As noted in Cynthia Klestinec, *Theaters of Anatomy: Students, Teachers, and Traditions of Dissection in Renaissance Venice* (Baltimore, MD, 2011), p. 34.
51 For the important relationship between clothes and status, see Giorgio Riello and Ulinka Rublack, eds, *The Right to Dress: Sumptuary Laws in a Global Perspective, c. 1200–1800* (Cambridge, 2019).
52 For the importance of the hand in anatomical literature, see further William Schupbach, *The Paradox of Rembrandt's 'Anatomy of Dr. Tulp'* (London, 1982), pp. 16–20, 57–65.
53 O'Malley, *Vesalius*, p. 148.

9 Making and Unmaking

1 *Fabrica*, p. 547. With the exception of Books Three and Four (on blood vessels and nerves), instructions for dissection are included at the end of each chapter.

2 Ibid., pp. 265–6 (scapula), 515–16 (kidney), 267 [367] (hemorrhoidal veins). See also Vivian Nutton, 'Montanus, Vesalius and the Haemorrhoidal Veins', *Clio Medica*, XVIII (1983), pp. 33–6.

3 G.E.R. Lloyd, *Polarity and Analogy: Two Types of Argumentation in Early Greek Thought* (Cambridge, 1966), pp. 285–94, 302–3; Margaret Tallmadge May, trans., *Galen: On the Usefulness of the Parts of the Body* (Ithaca, NY, 1968), vol. I, p. 159 (keel), vol. II, pp. 669 (house), 716 (woodcarvers); Charles Singer, trans., *Galen: On Anatomical Procedures*, repr. edn (Oxford, 1999), p. 158 (omentum). See also Bernadette Bensaude-Vincent and William R. Newman, eds, *The Artificial and the Natural: An Evolving Polarity* (Cambridge, 2007).

4 *Fabrica*, p. 592; Garrison and Hast, vol. II, p. 1198 (cited).

5 May, *Galen: On the Usefulness of the Parts*, vol. I, pp. 314–15; *Fabrica*, p. 592.

6 *Fabrica*, p. 633; Garrison and Hast, vol. II, pp. 1280–81 (cited).

7 These were also described (but not named) by Massa and Berengario, O'Malley, *Vesalius*, pp. 120–21.

8 *Fabrica*, pp. 15–16; Richardson and Carman, vol. I, p. 36 (cited in caption to illus. 68); compare Jacopo Berengario da Carpi, *Commentaria . . . super anatomia Mundini* (Bologna, 1521), fol. CCCCXVIIr (dovetailed joints).

9 *Fabrica*, pp. 154, 593.

10 Ibid., p. 291; Richardson and Carman, vol. II, p. 292 (cited). For the theme of 'Tennis and the Scientific Revolution', see *Nuncius*, XXVIII/1 (2013), special issue, ed. Marco Beretta and Alessandro Tosi.

11 *Fabrica*, pp. 578 (larynx), 242 [342] (pulley), and 344 [444] (cardinal's hat); Garrison and Hast, vol. I, p. 667, n. 44 for the hyaline cartilage covering the grooved surface of the ischium, vol. II, p. 900 (cited).

12 *Fabrica*, p. 225; Richardson and Carman, vol. II, p. 124 (cited).

13 As noted already in O'Malley, *Vesalius*, p. 141.

14 *Fabrica*, p. 39; Garrison and Hast, vol. I, p 84, n. 26, for the investment-casting process, 'cire perdue'. For Zoppo, see Victoria Avery, 'The Production, Display and Reception of Bronze Heads and Busts in Renaissance Venice and Padua: Surrogate Antiques', in *Kopf/Bild: Die Büste in Mittelalter und Früher Neuzeit*, ed. Jeanette Kohl and Rebecca Müller (Munich, 2007), pp. 75–112, at pp. 95–103.

15 *Fabrica*, pp. 646–7; Garrison and Hast, vol. II, p. 1307 (cited).
16 *Fabrica*, pp. 98, 624 (*fingeret*), 100 (*machinatur*), 340 [440] (*caelavit, insculpserit*), 500 (*formari*), 518 (*efformavit*), 578 (*creatus sit*), 600 (*artificium*), 53, 59, 193 (*industria*), 122 (*non minimam solertiam*), 493, 555, 596 (*providentia*).
17 Ibid., pp. 88 (*Opificis rerum in thorace creandi industria*), 240 (*Conditor*), 569 (*architectus*), 583 (*summus rerum Opifex*).
18 Ibid., pp. 65, 225 [325] (*inartificiosissimam constructionem*); Garrison and Hast, vol. I, pp. 132, 636 (cited).
19 *Fabrica*, p. 341 [441]; Garrison and Hast, vol. II, p. 893, n. 14.
20 *Fabrica*, pp. 234 (membrane), 230 [330], 462 [262] (scapula), 550 (bladder).
21 For example, ibid., pp. 275, 300, 254 [354].
22 Ibid., p. 564; Garrison and Hast, vol. II, p. 1215 (cited in caption to illus. 69, my insertion).
23 *Fabrica*, pp. 274 [374], 556, 601, 658.
24 Ibid., p. 39.
25 Ibid., pp. 278, 223 [323], 603.
26 Ibid., p. 274; Richardson and Carman, vol. II, 247 (cited).
27 *Fabrica*, p. 236 [336].
28 Ibid., p. 274.
29 Ibid., p. 275 [375].
30 Ibid., pp. 260, 548, 556.
31 Ibid., p. 269.
32 Ibid., p. 260; Richardson and Carman, vol. II, p. 214 (cited).
33 *Fabrica*, p. 507; Richardson and Carman, vol. IV, p. 109 (cited).
34 This section summarizes *Fabrica*, pp. 155–62; Richardson and Carman, vol. I, p. 378 (cited in caption to illus. 70).
35 Charles Zika, *The Appearance of Witchcraft: Images and Social Meaning in 16th-Century Europe* (London, 2007), pp. 70–98.
36 *Fabrica*, p. 159; Richardson and Carman, vol. I, p. 378 (cited).
37 *Fabrica*, p. 209; Richardson and Carman, vol. II, p. 91 (cited).
38 *Fabrica*, p. 159; Garrison and Hast, vol. I, p. 310 (cited).
39 Suzanne Karr Schmidt, *Interactive and Sculptural Printmaking in the Renaissance* (Leiden, 2017), pp. 127–9, records only twelve surviving copies where the constructed manikins are intact.
40 Tim Huisman, *The Finger of God: Anatomical Practice in 17th-Century Leiden* (Leiden, 2009), pp. 17–42.
41 *Fabrica*, pp. 283, 602.

10 After *Fabrica*

1   For biographical details in this chapter, I follow O'Malley, *Vesalius*,
    pp. 189–282; and Maurits Biesrouck, 'Andreas Vesalius's Fatal
    Voyage to Jerusalem (4)', *Medical Terminology* (16 June 2016), https://
    clinicalanatomy.com/mtd/806. For the presentation copy, see Diana
    H. Hook and Jeremy M. Norman, *The Haskell F. Norman Library of
    Science and Medicine* (San Francisco, 1991), vol. II, pp. 779–80 (no.
    2137), plates XXVII–XXIX.

2   O'Malley, *Vesalius*, pp. 194–5, 240–44, 255–6, 431, n. 45; F.A.F.T.
    Reiffenberg, ed., *Lettres sur la vie intérieur de l'empereur Charles-Quint, écrites
    par Guillaume van Male* (Brussels, 1843), p. 74; Henry de Vocht, ed.,
    Literae Virorum eruditorum ad Franciscum Craneveldium 1522–1528,
    Humanistica Lovaniensia, I (Louvain, 1928), p. 536; Omer Steeno
    and Maurits Biesbrouck, 'Esquisse biographique de Nicola(us)
    Florenas mentor d'André Vésale', *Vesalius – Acta Internationalia Historiae
    Medicinae*, XVIII/I (2012), pp. 16–17.

3   Cornelis van Baersdorp, *Methodus universae artis medicae* (Bruges, 1538),
    with a woodcut title page.

4   Vivian Nutton, 'Renaissance Galenism, 1540–1640: Flexibility or an
    Increasing Irrelevance?', in *Brill's Companion to the Reception of Galen*, ed.
    Petros Bouras-Vallianatos and Barbara Zipser (Leiden, 2019),
    pp. 472–86.

5   John M. Forrester, 'The Marvellous Network and the History of
    Enquiry into Its Function', *Journal of the History of Medicine and Allied
    Sciences*, LVII (2002), pp. 198–217.

6   Jacobo Facciolati, ed., *Fasti gymnasii Patavini: Ab anno* MDXVII *ad*
    MDCCLVI (Padua, 1757), pp. 337–8, 343, 386.

7   D. H. Garrison, trans., *Andreas Vesalius: The China Root Epistle: A New
    Translation and Critical Edition* (Cambridge, 2015), pp. 47–52; Anna E.
    Winterbottom, 'Of the China Root: A Case Study of the Early
    Modern Circulation of Materia Medica', *Social History of Medicine*,
    XXVIII/I (2015), pp. 22–44, at p. 23.

8   O'Malley, *Vesalius*, pp. 385–6; Sachiko Kusukawa, *Picturing the Book of
    Nature: Image, Text, and Argument in Sixteenth-Century Human Anatomy and
    Medical Botany* (Chicago, IL, 2012), pp. 135–6.

9   Wolfgang Klose and Wolfgang Harms, eds, *Wittenberger
    Gelehrtenstammbuch: Das Stammbuch von Abraham und David Ulrich, benutzt
    von 1549–1577 sowie 1580–1623*, 2 vols (Halle, 1999), vol. I, pp. 24–5,
    226, vol. II (facsimile), p. 412 (fol. 145v). I thank Professor Iain
    Donaldson for drawing my attention to this material. For the

Lutheran origin of such collections of autographs, see Ulinka Rublack, 'Grapho-Relics: Lutheranism and the Materialization of the Word', in *Relics and Remains*, ed. A. Walsham (Oxford, 2010), pp. 144–66.

10 O'Malley, *Vesalius*, pp. 196, 205–6, 230.

11 Vivian Nutton, 'Vesalius Revised: His Annotations to the 1555 *Fabrica*', *Medical History*, LVI/4 (October 2012), pp. 415–43.

12 As translated in Charles D. O'Malley, 'Andreas Vesalius, Count Palatine: Further Information on Vesalius and His Ancestors', *Journal of the History of Medicine and Allied Sciences*, IX/2 (1954), pp. 196–223, at p. 207.

13 For diplomatic gifts, see Zoltán Biedermann, Anne Gerritsen and Giorgio Riello, eds, *Global Gifts: The Material Culture of Diplomacy in Early Modern Eurasia* (Cambridge, 2017).

14 I summarize here O'Malley, *Vesalius*, pp. 283–8, 296–302.

15 This paragraph is based on ibid., pp. 378–402.

16 Garrison, *China Root*, p. 45; O'Malley, *Vesalius*, p. 379.

17 Facciolati, *Fasti*, p. 387.

18 This paragraph is based on Gabriele Falloppio, *Observationes anatomicae* (Venice, 1561), fols 1r–2r (Vesalius and Galen), 2v (*anatomicum, philosophum, medicum*), 20v, 25r, 55v, 121v, 125r, 147r, 172r (*divinus Vesalius*), 26v–30v (ear), 65v–66v (eyelid), 80v (*veritas*), 197r (*tuba*); Cynthia Klestinec, *Theaters of Anatomy: Students, Teachers, and Traditions of Dissection in Renaissance Venice* (Baltimore, MD, 2011), pp. 42–54; Ian Maclean, 'Vesalius as Authority: From the First Publications to the Opera Omnia of 1725', in *Towards the Authority of Vesalius: Studies on Medicine and the Human Body from Antiquity to the Renaissance and Beyond*, ed. Erika Gielen and Michèle Goyens (Turnhout, 2018), pp. 23–47, at pp. 33–5.

19 Andreas Vesalius, *Anatomicarum Gabrielis Falloppii observationum examen* (Venice, 1564), p. 171, as noted in Andrew Cunningham, *The Anatomical Renaissance: The Resurrection of the Anatomical Projects of the Ancients* (Aldershot, 1997), p. 121. See also Harvey W. Cushing, *A Bio-Bibliography of Andreas Vesalius* (New York, 1943), pp. 182–94.

20 This paragraph is based on Dániel Margócsy, Mark Somos and Stephen N. Joffe, eds, *The Fabrica of Andreas Vesalius: A Worldwide Descriptive Census, Ownership, and Annotations of the 1543 and 1555 Editions* (Leiden, 2018), pp. 30–37, 56–106, 360–61.

21 Galen, *Opera Omnia* (Venice, 1542), vol. I, cols 418, 428, 441, 446, 462, 519, 550, 614, 662, 698, 762, John Rylands Library, the University of Manchester, RR 221882.

22 Margaret Tallmadge May, trans., *Galen: On the Usefulness of the Parts of the Body* (Ithaca, NY, 1968), vol. I, p. 115 (cited in caption to illus. 72); *Fabrica*, p. 172.

23 For copies of Vesalius's work, a helpful start is still Cushing, *A Bio-Bibliography of Andreas Vesalius*, pp. 119-53. For the meaning of copying to modern times, see Dániel Margócsy, 'From Vesalius through Ivins to Latour: Imitation, Emulation and Exactly Repeatable Pictorial Statements in the *Fabrica*', *Word and Image*, XXXV/3 (2019), pp. 315–33.

24 This paragraph draws on Thomas Geminus, *Compendiosa totius anatomie delineatio, ære exarata* (London, 1545), fol. [2]r; Peter Murray Jones, 'Gemini [Geminus, Lambrit], Thomas (fl. 1540–1562), engraver, printer and instrument maker', *Oxford Dictionary of National Biography*, 2004, online edition, www.oxforddnb.com; Alexander Sampson, 'Mapping the Marriage: Thomas Geminus's "Britanniae Insulae Nova Descriptio" and "Nova Descriptio Hispaniae" (1555)', *Renaissance and Reformation*, XXXI/1 (2008), pp. 95–115, especially p. 103; Melissa Lo, 'Cut, Copy and English Anatomy: Thomas Geminus and the Reordering of Vesalius's Canonical Body', in *Andreas Vesalius and the Fabrica in the Age of Printing: Art, Anatomy and Printing in the Italian Renaissance*, ed. Rinaldo F. Canalis and Massimo Ciavolella (Turnhout, 2018), pp. 226–56.

25 Thomas Geminus, *Compendiosa totius anatomie delineatio, ære exarata* (London, 1553), fol. [2]v.

26 Duncan P. Thomas, 'Thomas Vicary and the *Anatomie of Mans Body*', *Medical History*, L (2006), pp. 235–46.

27 Ruth Mortimer, *Harvard College Library, Department of Printing and Graphic Arts: Catalogue of Books and Manuscripts; French 16th Century Books* (Cambridge, MA, 1964), vol. II, p. 661 (no. 541).

28 Vesalius, *Epitome* (Paris, 1560), p. [144].

29 Jacques Grévin, *Anatomes totius, aere insculpta delineatio* (Paris, 1564), fols *ijr–v.

30 Jacques Grévin, *Les Portraicts anatomiques de toutes les parties du corps humain* (Paris, 1569), fols *ijr–v; Jacqueline Vons, 'Jacques Grévin (1538–1570) et la nomenclature anatomique française', in *Lire, choisir, écrire*, ed. Violaine Giacomotto-Charra and Christine Silvi (Paris, 2014), pp. 133–48.

31 Juan de Valverde, *Historia de la composicion del cuerpo humano* (Rome, 1556), fols *ijr–v. I also draw on Bjørn Okholm Skaarup, 'The Unexpected Success of a Spanish Anatomy Book: Juan Valverde de Amusco's *Historia de la composicion del cuerpo humano* (Rome, 1556), and

Its Many Later Editions', in *Specialist Markets in the Early Modern Book World*, ed. Richard Kirwan and Sophie Mullins (Leiden, 2015), pp. 123–41.

32 Valverde, *Historia*, fol. [*iii]r.

33 Juan de Valverde, *Anatomia del corpo humano* (Rome, 1559), fol. a2r.

34 Cunningham, *Anatomical Renaissance*, pp. 143–66.

35 Leon Voet, *The Plantin Press (1555–1589): A Bibliography of the Works Printed and Published by Christopher Plantin at Antwerp and Leiden* (Amsterdam, 1980), vol. v, pp. 2328–33 (no. 2413).

36 *Vivae imagines partium corporis humani aereis formis expressae* (Antwerp, 1566), fols A2r–A3r.

37 Shizu Sakai, trans., *Kaitai shinsho: Zen gendaigo yaku* (Tokyo, 1998).

38 For the 1725 edition, see Margócsy, 'From Vesalius through Ivins to Latour', pp. 326–9; Maclean, 'Vesalius as Authority', pp. 40–42.

SELECT BIBLIOGRAPHY

Digital Sites

A list of digitized copies of *Fabrica* (both editions) is available at the site of the Vesalius Census, www.vesaliuscensus.com/digital-fabricas. Other rare historical books mentioned in this book may be found at the site of Bibliothèque numérique Medica (Bibliothèques d'Université Paris Cité), www.biusante.parisdescartes.fr/histoire/medica, or the Bavarian State Library, Munich, www.digitale-sammlungen.de/en.

A comprehensive bibliography of studies about Vesalius is available at a site maintained by Maurits Biesbrouck, with additional information at www.andreasvesalius.be or https://fatherofanatomy.wordpress.com.

Translations of Original Texts

Eriksson, Ruben, trans., *Andreas Vesalius' First Public Anatomy at Bologna 1540: An Eyewitness Report by Baldasar Heseler* (Uppsala and Stockholm, 1959) [Eriksson, *Eyewitness* in references]

Garrison, Daniel H., trans., *Vesalius: The China Root Epistle: A New Translation and Critical Edition* (Cambridge, 2015)

—, and Malcolm Howard Hast, trans., *The Fabric of the Human Body: An Annotated Translation of the 1543 and 1555 Editions of 'De Humani Corporis Fabrica Libri Septem'*, 2 vols (Basle, 2014) [Garrison and Hast in references]

Lind, Levi Robert, trans., *A Short Introduction to Anatomy – Isagoge Breves by Jacopo Berengario da Carpi* (Chicago, IL, 1959)

—, trans., *Studies in Pre-Vesalian Anatomy: Biography, Translations, Documents* (Philadelphia, PA, 1975)

—, trans., *On Fracture of the Skull or Cranium by Jacopo Berengario da Carpi* (Philadelphia, PA, 1990)

May, Margaret Tallmadge, trans., *Galen: On the Usefulness of the Parts of the Body*, 2 vols (Ithaca, NY, 1968)

Nutton, Vivian, ed. and trans., *Principles of Anatomy according to the Opinion of Galen by Johann Guinter and Andreas Vesalius* (London, 2017)

Richardson, William Frank, and John Burd Carman, trans., *On the Fabric of the Human Body: A Translation of 'De Humani Corporis Fabrica Libri Septem'*, 5 vols (San Francisco, CA, 1998–2009) [Richardson and Carman in references]

Singer, Charles, trans., *Galen: On Anatomical Procedures*, repr. edn (Oxford, 1999)

Vons, Jacqueline, trans., and Stéphane Velut, *Résumé de ses livres sur la fabrique du corps* (Paris, 2008)

Studies on Vesalius

Canalis, Rinaldo F., and Massimo Ciavolella, eds, *Andreas Vesalius and the Fabrica in the Age of Printing: Art, Anatomy and Printing in the Italian Renaissance* (Turnhout, 2018)

Carlino, Andrea, *Books of the Body: Anatomical Ritual and Renaissance Learning*, trans. John Tedeschi and Anne C. Tedeschi (Chicago, IL, 1999)

Cunningham, Andrew, *The Anatomical Renaissance: The Resurrection of the Anatomical Projects of the Ancients* (Aldershot, 1997)

Cushing, Harvey W., ed., *A Bio-Bibliography of Andreas Vesalius* (New York, NY, 1943)

Gielen, Erika, and Michèle Goyens, eds, *Towards the Authority of Vesalius: Studies on Medicine and the Human Body from Antiquity to the Renaissance and Beyond* (Turnhout, 2018)

Harcourt, Glenn, 'Andreas Vesalius and the Anatomy of Antique Sculpture', *Representations*, XVII (1987), pp. 28–61

Kornell, Monique, 'Jan Steven van Calcar, c. 1515–c. 1546, Vesalius' Illustrator', in *Andreas Vesalius and the Fabrica in the Age of Printing: Art, Anatomy and Printing in the Italian Renaissance*, ed. Rinaldo F. Canalis and Massimo Ciavolella (Turnhout, 2018), pp. 99–130

Lambert, Samuel W., Willy Wiegand and William W. Ivins Jr, *Three Vesalian Essays to Accompany the Icones Anatomicae of 1934* (New York, NY, 1952)

Maclean, Ian, 'Vesalius as Authority: From the First Publications to the Opera Omnia of 1725', in *Towards the Authority of Vesalius: Studies on Medicine and the Human Body from Antiquity to the Renaissance and Beyond*, ed. Erika Gielen and Michèle Goyens (Turnhout, 2018), pp. 23–47

Margócsy, Dániel, Mark Somos and Stephen N. Joffe, eds, *The Fabrica of Andreas Vesalius: A Worldwide Descriptive Census, Ownership, and Annotations of the 1543 and 1555 Editions* (Leiden, 2018)

O'Malley, Charles D., *Andreas Vesalius of Bårussels, 1514–1564* (Berkeley, CA, 1964) [O'Malley, *Vesalius* in references]

Siraisi, Nancy G., 'Vesalius and Human Diversity in *De Humani Corporis Fabrica*', *Journal of the Warburg and Courtauld Institutes*, LVII (1994), pp. 60–88

—, 'Vesalius and the Reading of Galen's Teleology', *Renaissance Quarterly*, L/1 (1997), pp. 1–37

Other Related Studies

Bouras-Vallianatos, Petros, and Barbara Zipser, eds, *Brill's Companion to the Reception of Galen* (Leiden, 2019)

Bylebyl, Jerome J., 'The School of Padua: Humanistic Medicine in the Sixteenth Century', in *Health, Medicine and Mortality in the Sixteenth Century*, ed. Charles Webster (Cambridge, 1979), pp. 335–70

Grendler, Paul F., *The Universities of the Italian Renaissance* (Baltimore, MD, 2002)

Kemp, Martin, *Leonardo da Vinci: The Marvellous Works of Nature and Man*, revd edn (Oxford, 2006)

Klestinec, Cynthia, *Theaters of Anatomy: Students, Teachers, and Traditions of Dissection in Renaissance Venice* (Baltimore, MD, 2011)

Kornell, Monique, Erin Travers, Thisbe Gensler and Naoko Takahatake, *Flesh and Bones: The Art of Anatomy*, exh. cat., Getty Museum, Los Angeles (2022)

Kusukawa, Sachiko, *Picturing the Book of Nature: Image, Text, and Argument in Sixteenth-Century Human Anatomy and Medical Botany* (Chicago, IL, 2012)

McKitterick, David, *Print, Manuscript and the Search for Order, 1450–1830* (Cambridge, 2003)

Maclean, Ian, *Logic, Signs and Nature: Learned Medicine in the Renaissance* (Cambridge, 2001)

—, *Learning and the Market Place: Essays in the History of the Early Modern Book* (Leiden, 2009)

Margócsy, Dániel, 'From Vesalius through Ivins to Latour: Imitation, Emulation and Exactly Repeatable Pictorial Statements in the *Fabrica*', *Word and Image*, XXXV/3 (2019), pp. 315–33

Martin, Henri-Jean, and Jean Vezin, eds, *Mise en page et mise en texte du livre manuscrit* (Paris, 1990)

Nova, Alessandro, and Domenico Laurenza, eds, *Leonardo da Vinci's Anatomical World* (Venice, 2011)

Nutton, Vivian, *Ancient Medicine* (London, 2004)

Park, Katharine, 'The Criminal and the Saintly Body: Autopsy and Dissection in Renaissance Italy', *Renaissance Quarterly*, XLVII/1 (1994), pp. 1–33

—, *Secrets of Women: Gender, Generation, and the Origins of Human Dissection* (New York, NY, 2006)

Siraisi, Nancy G., *Medieval and Early Renaissance Medicine: An Introduction to Knowledge and Practice* (Chicago, IL, 1990)

Wagner, Bettina, ed., *Worlds of Learning: The Library and World Chronicle of the Nuremberg Physician Hartmann Schedel (1440–1514)*, trans. Diane Booton and Bettina Wagner, exh. cat., Bavarian State Library, Munich (2015)

Wear, Andrew, R. K. French and Iain M. Lonie, eds, *The Medical Renaissance of the Sixteenth Century* (Cambridge, 1985)

ACKNOWLEDGEMENTS

This book, like any study on Vesalius, owes an immense debt to the seminal works of Charles D. O'Malley as well as to the translators of the modern editions, John Burd Carman, Daniel Garrison, Malcolm Hast, Willliam F. Richardson and Jacqueline Vons. Critical for writing this book were also the insights of Jerome Bylebyl, Glenn Harcourt, Martin Kemp, Ian Maclean, Vivian Nutton, Richard Palmer, Katharine Park and Nancy Siraisi. I am especially indebted to Andrew Cunningham, whose lectures on the Renaissance and Vesalius many years ago were an inspiration and the starting point of my own fascination with both topics, and who kindly commented on a draft of this book. Nick Jardine, Dániel Margócsy, François Quiviger, Ulinka Rublack and the late Iain Donaldson also offered encouragement, corrections and comments for improvements on earlier versions of this book. A chance meeting in May 2023 revealed that Vivian Nutton was also writing a book on Vesalius. I am grateful to him for generously sharing with me an early draft of his forthcoming book, *Changing the World of Anatomy. Andreas Vesalius and his 'Fabrica'*, though I was unable to benefit fully from his findings, as my book was already in production.

In writing this book, I have benefited from the support of friends and colleagues. I am particularly grateful to Alexandra Walsham for her unfailing kindness, wisdom and good sense. For their encouragement and advice, I thank Monica Azzolini, Catherine Barnard, Annabel Brett, Lorraine Daston, Sven Dupré, Florike Egmond, Moti Feingold, Paula Findlen, Sietske Fransen, Marina Frasca Spada, Sian Gardner, Roger Gaskell, Lynn Gladden, Takehiko Hashimoto, Tamara Hug, Peter Murray Jones, Eric Jorink, Monique Kornell, Elaine Leong, Karin Leonhard, Evelyn Lincoln, David McKitterick, Scott Mandelbrote, Alexander Marr, Peter Mason, Lea Olsan, Katharine Park, Richard Ratzan, Eileen Reeves, Katherine Reinhart, Joan Richards, Martin Rudwick, Daniel Sherman, Emma Spary, the late Christine Salazar, Richard Serjeantson, Claudia Stein, Liba Taub, Teresa Webber, the late Frances

Willmoth and Grae Worster. They reminded me that I was not writing in a vacuum.

I am also grateful for the assistance I received from Helga Tichy at the Bavarian State Library; Dr Emily Dourish and Claire Welford at the Department of Rare Books and Johanna Ward at the Digital Content Unit at Cambridge University Library; Steven Hartshorne at John Rylands Library, University of Manchester; Dr Anne Rothfeld and Krista R. Stracka at the National Library of Medicine, Bethesda; Kate Symmonds at the Wellcome Library; and Dr Nicolas Bell, Steven Archer and James Kirwan at the Wren Library.

I thank Michael Leaman, Alex Ciobanu, Susannah Jayes, Emma Devlin and their team at Reaktion for their patience in seeing this book through to production.

Hiroko Kusukawa, Noriko Kusukawa, Carl Wittwer and Tori Wittwer Kusukawa have kept me grounded with perspective and light relief while my husband, Keith Ball, as always, has been immensely supportive, patient and understanding. This book is for my father, Toru Kusukawa, who died before its completion. He taught me many things and enabled me to pursue an unusual career for a Japanese daughter.

PHOTO ACKNOWLEDGEMENTS

The author and publishers wish to express their thanks to the sources listed below for illustrative material and/or permission to reproduce it. Some locations of artworks are also given below, in the interest of brevity:

Bayersiche Staatsbibliothek, Munich: 6 (Clm 363, fol. 170v), 7 (Clm 363, fol. 107r), 8 (Clm 168, fol. 116v), 10 (2 Inc.c.a.3216, fol. 16r), 11 (2 Inc.c.a.3216, fol. 28v), 12 (Rar.287, fol. XLIIIv), 23 (Med.g. 517, a7r), 56 (Rar. 747#Beibd.1, scan 14), 57 (Rar. 747#Beibd.1, scan 15), 58 (Rar. 747#Beibd.1, scan 26), 59 (Rar. 747#Beibd.1, scan 27); Biblioteca Nazionale Marciana, Venice (228.d.1, c.16), photos reproduced with the permission of the Italian Ministry of Culture, all rights reserved: 24, 25; British Library, London (Harley MS 2726, fol. 194v), photo © British Library Board, all rights reserved/Bridgeman Images: 9; Cambridge University Library (CCF.46.36), photos reproduced by kind permission of the Syndics of Cambridge University Library: 3, 4, 5, 35, 53; Cambridge University Library (N*.1.1(A)), photo reproduced by kind permission of the Syndics of Cambridge University Library: 71; Cambridge University Library (N*.1.2(A)), photos reproduced by kind permission of the Syndics of Cambridge University Library: 1, 26, 29, 30, 31, 33, 34, 38, 39, 40, 41, 42, 43, 45, 46, 47, 48, 49, 50, 51, 52, 54, 55, 60, 61, 62, 63, 64, 65, 66, 67, 68, 69, 70; Cambridge University Library (N*.13.7(B)), photo reproduced by kind permission of the Syndics of Cambridge University Library: 32; Crocker Art Museum, Sacramento, CA (E. B. Crocker Collection, 1871.127): 28; © Kupferstichkabinett, Staatliche Museen zu Berlin: 2; The Master and Fellows of Trinity College, Cambridge: 13 (Grylls. II. 403), 44 (S.5.6); National Diet Library, Tokyo: 75; National Library of Medicine, Bethesda, MD: 27; © Österreichische Nationalbibliothek, Vienna: 14 (68.G.39, fol. ev recto); Royal Collection Trust/© His Majesty King Charles III 2023: 36; © The Trustees of the British Museum: 37; © The University of Manchester: 72; Wellcome Collection, London: 15, 16, 17, 18, 19, 20, 21, 22, 73, 74.

INDEX

Illustration numbers are indicated by *italics*